Fine Needle Aspiration of the Breast

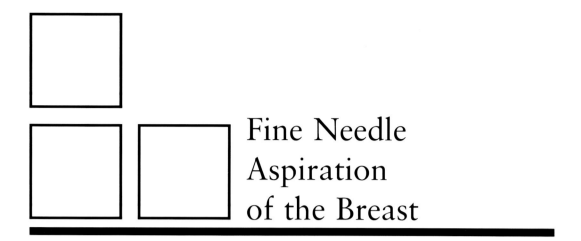

Fine Needle Aspiration of the Breast

YOLANDA C. OERTEL, M.D.

Professor of Pathology
The George Washington University School of Medicine
Washington, D.C.

Butterworths

Boston   London   Durban   Singapore   Sydney   Toronto   Wellington

Library of Congress Cataloging-in-Publication Data

Oertel, Yolanda C.
  Fine needle aspiration of the breast.

  Bibliography: p.
  1. Breast—Biopsy, Needle. 2. Breast—Diseases—
Diagnosis. 3. Breast—Cancer—Diagnosis. 4. Diagnosis,
Cytologic. I. Title. [DNLM: 1. Biopsy, Needle.
2. Breast Diseases—diagnosis. 3. Breast Neoplasms—
diagnosis. WP 815 O29f]
RG493.5.B56037   618.1'907'58   86—28405
ISBN 0—409—95192—7

Butterworth Publishers
80 Montvale Avenue
Stoneham, MA 02180

10 9 8 7 6 5 4 3 2 1

Printed in the United States of America

To the memory of William Newman, M.D., former Director of Anatomic Pathology and Professor of Pathology, The George Washington University Medical Center. With respect and gratitude to an expert diagnostician who contributed to my training and who exemplified service and concern for the patient.

Contents

Preface   xi

Acknowledgments   xiii

1. INTRODUCTION   1

2. ADVANTAGES AND DISADVANTAGES OF FINE NEEDLE ASPIRATION   4
   Advantages for the Patient   4
   Advantages for the Surgeon and/or Internist   5
   Advantages for the Hospital   6
   Advantages for the Pathologist   6
   Disadvantages of Fine Needle Aspiration: Real and Theoretical   6
   Complications   7
   Needle Biopsies   7

3. QUESTIONS ASKED MOST FREQUENTLY   8
   Why Diff-Quik?   8
   How Did We Get Started?   10
   The Patient and Informed Consent   11
   The Aspiration Team in the Pathology Department   12
   The Aspiration Room   13
   The Crux of the Matter   14

4. **FINE NEEDLE ASPIRATION TECHNIQUE**   16
    What Is Needed to Perform an Aspiration?   16
    How to Perform the Aspiration   19
    Preparation of the Smears   22
    Staining of the Smears   25
    How to Learn to Perform the Procedure   28

5. **HOW TO SUCCEED AT FINE NEEDLE ASPIRATION**   29
    What Is an Adequate Sample?   30
    Unsatisfactory Specimens   31
    Reasons for Unsatisfactory Specimens   31
    Why Is a Particular Aspiration Performed?   32

6. **USUAL FINDINGS IN THE ASPIRATES**   34
    Adipose Tissue   34
    Normal Ductal Cells   34
    Myoepithelial Cells   38
    Stripped Nuclei   38
    Apocrine Metaplastic Cells   38
    Histiocytes   39
    Oleic Acid Crystals   44
    Breast Lobules   44

7. **OCCASIONAL FINDINGS IN THE ASPIRATES**   45
    Skeletal Muscle   45
    Skin   45
    Platelets   45
    Microcalcifications   49
    Artifacts   49

8. **BENIGN LESIONS**   56
    Non-neoplastic Disorders   56
    Lesions Secondary to Trauma   68
    Hormonal Changes   68
    Bacterial and Viral Diseases   71
    Benign Neoplasms   78
    Miscellaneous   89

9. **ATYPICAL DUCTAL HYPERPLASIA**   94
    Ductal Hyperplasia or Atypical Ductal Hyperplasia?   94
    Ductal Hyperplasia or Neoplasia?   101
    Atypical Ductal Hyperplasia or Neoplasia?   103

10. **GENERAL DIAGNOSTIC CRITERIA OF MALIGNANCY**   104
    Infiltration   108

Nucleus   108
Intranuclear Inclusions or Vacuoles   108
Nucleolus   108
Intracellular or Intracytoplasmic Lumina   109
Mitotic Figures   111
Blood Vessels   111

11. ADENOCARCINOMAS   112
Ductal Adenocarcinomas   112
Relatively Rare Ductal Carcinomas   124
Lobular Carcinoma   145
Carcinoma in Unusual Hosts   149

12. MALIGNANT NONEPITHELIAL NEOPLASMS   150
Leukemia and Lymphoma   150
Mycosis Fungoides   150
Cystosarcoma Phyllodes   155

13. METASTATIC TUMORS IN THE BREAST   156
Malignant Melanoma   156
Renal Cell Carcinoma   158

14. THORACIC WALL RECURRENCES AND AXILLARY MASSES   161
Axillary Lymph Node Metastases   161
Neoplasms of Nervous Tissue   165
Accessory Mammary Tissue in Axilla   166

15. PITFALLS   167
Organizing Hematoma   167
Herpetic Infection of the Nipple   167
Granular Cell Tumor Versus Ductal Ectasia   168
Fat Necrosis   170
Comedomastitis   171
Acute Mastitis and Abscess   171
Fibroadenomas   174
Radiation-Induced Atypia   179
Misconceptions   181

16. FINE NEEDLE ASPIRATION OF NONPALPABLE BREAST LESIONS   182

17. ADDITIONAL DIAGNOSTIC INFORMATION   184
Consistency of Lesion when Needling   184
Appearance of Smears with the Naked Eye   185
Guidelines for Smear Examination   185
General Reminders   185

18. **STATISTICAL SUMMARY**   187
     False Negatives and False Positives   190
     Inconclusive Aspirates   194

References   197

Index   201

Preface

Fine needle aspiration is a valuable diagnostic tool that is gaining increased acceptance in the United States. It helps clinicians and surgeons arrive at a more correct diagnosis in a timely and economical fashion and enhances their ability to manage patients effectively.

This monograph is intended for practicing surgical pathologists and pathology residents and fellows who are interested in getting started or have little or no practical experience with fine needle aspiration of the breast.

Based on my experience at a 500-bed university hospital during the last nine years, I believe, like the Scandinavians, that (1) better results are obtained when the pathologist performs the aspirations, and that (2) it is easier to interpret hematologically stained smears. For these reasons we emphasize the technical aspects of the procedure; all our diagnostic criteria and the illustrations of this monograph are from smears stained with Diff-Quik (see Chapter 3 for the reasons we chose this stain).

I discuss only entities with which I have had personal experience. Due to limitations of space, I have omitted any photographs of histologic sections. I assume that the reader has a background in surgical pathology. If not, he or she would find it difficult to master fine needle aspiration because a thorough knowledge of the pathologic processes in tissues is needed to understand the spectrum of cellular changes observed in the smears.

I have been selective of references and have included only those which in my opinion are the most useful ones. This reflects my personal choice or bias.

I hope this effort will prove useful to the surgical pathologist and that it will stimulate interest in fine needle aspiration.

Y.C.O.

Acknowledgments

In the spring of 1980 the American Society of Clinical Pathologists (ASCP) gave me the opportunity to present a workshop titled "Fine Needle Aspiration: A Diagnostic Tool." Two years later it was expanded to an Educational Center Program, and thus required further review and organization of my cases. The pathologists attending these workshops asked many questions and desired clear diagnostic criteria. Without that initial stimulus from the ASCP, I could not have attempted to write this monograph.

I am grateful to my staff for their dedication and continuous efforts to provide good service to patients and physicians. I am particularly grateful to Miss Mayo Mendoza, CT(ASCP), for her loyalty and commitment to excellence, and to Mrs. Carolyn McCauley for her organizational abilities and untiring typing. In addition, I would like to acknowledge the help of Miss L. Poprocky CT(ASCP), and Mrs. K. Webb, CT(ASCP), for performing whatever duty was necessary with their usual pleasantness.

My special thanks go to Kersti Hedberg, M.D., who taught me how to perform the fine needle aspiration and whose aspiration service at Sahlgrenska Sjukhuset has served as my blueprint.

My thanks to the staff of The George Washington University Medical Center Audiovisual Services and in particular to Ms. Barbara Neuberger for her continuous help with the photomicrographs.

My gratitude to Mr. Robert du Treil, Jr. (The George Washington University School of Engineering) for his enormous help with the IBM–XT.

Many surgeons and internists have contributed follow-up information on their patients. Among the most helpful physicians and their staffs I would like to acknowledge Drs. K. Alley, A. Baer, J. Canter, M. Cohen, R. Flax, R. Kurstin,

H. Tidler, and Mrs. E. Mabry and Mrs. B. Stewart of the Group Health Association. I would also like to thank the pathology departments of the following institutions for providing histologic follow-up: Holy Cross Hospital and Cytology Services, both of Silver Spring, MD; the National Institutes of Health, Bethesda, MD; Washington Hospital Center, Columbia Hospital for Women, and Georgetown University Hospital, all of Washington DC; and Fairfax Hospital and Arlington Hospital, both of Virginia.

There are some individuals who although no longer associated with The George Washington University Medical Center have helped me along the way. R. Malmgren, M.D., was instrumental in getting me started with fine needle aspiration, and L.I. Galblum, M.D., collaborated with me in a previous publication that became the backbone for this monograph.

Last, but not least, my gratitude to my husband, J. E. Oertel, M.D., for his tolerance, support, and critical editorial assistance.

Fine Needle
Aspiration
of the Breast

Introduction

The procedure that we will address is fine needle aspiration, referred to by some pathologists as fine needle aspiration *biopsy*. This latter term is confusing for several reasons:

1. The material obtained is cellular material, which is then smeared on glass slides. When tissue fragments are obtained, they are so small that they are crushed on the slide and no special processing is required prior to examination.
2. In needle biopsies or "true-cut biopsies" a tissue core is obtained that has to be processed to paraffin or plastic prior to sectioning with a microtome. The sections are then stained with hematoxylin and eosin before microscopic diagnosis.
3. The largest needle we use for aspirations is 22-gauge. Compare it to the diameter of a Silverman needle used for biopsies (Fig. 1.1).
4. More and more pathologists are going to perform this procedure, and I would like to make their task a little easier. Biopsies, as a rule, are obtained by surgeons. Hence, when a patient comes to the pathologist for a "biopsy," she questions this, and the pathologist has to spend time explaining that it is not really a biopsy but just an aspiration.
5. To perform a needle biopsy, anesthesia usually is required. This is not the case with fine needle aspiration.
6. Consideration also should be given to the additional payment required for professional liability insurance when performing "needle biopsies" because they are classified as "minor surgery." Needle aspirations are not considered minor surgery.

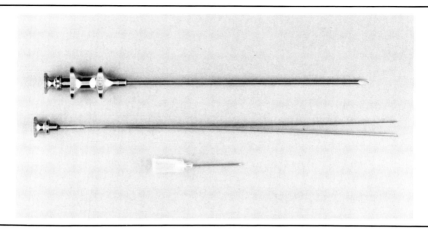

Figure 1.1.
Silverman biopsy needle (with stylet) and split needle. Needle for aspiration with clear plastic hub (22-gauge).

Figure 1.2.
Number of fine needle aspirations performed yearly at The George Washington University Medical Center from 1976 through 1984.

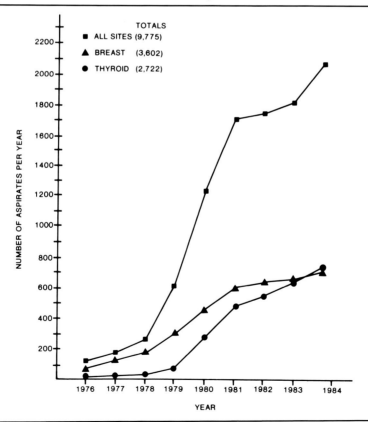

What follows is the product of our experience in the last nine years, in which we have interpreted and/or performed close to 10,000 aspirates (Fig. 1.2), of which 3,570 were aspirations from palpable, solid masses of the breast and 32 were from lesions detected only by mammograms. We emphasize the solid nature of the lesions because in our laboratory the fluid aspirated from mammary cysts is processed and counted with the rest of the nongynecologic material, such as ascitic fluid, pleural fluid, *etc.* Most of the fluids from breast cysts are submitted by surgeons and gynecologists. However, also classified as aspirations are smears from a lesion remaining after removal of fluid; of course, if we included the fluids from cysts we easily could add 3,000 more cases to this series. Except for three cases, smears from nipple discharges have not been included.

The history of fine needle aspiration has been reviewed in previous publications (Webb 1974, pp. 62−64; Rush 1977, pp. 33−34; Frable 1983, pp. 2−4; Koss et al. 1984, pp. 3−5; Feldman and Covell 1985, pp. 3−4). Four papers merit particular attention: the two classic publications of Martin and Ellis (1930 and 1934), the one by Stewart (1933), and an editorial by Koss (1980).

Although not directly related to fine needle aspiration, the reader might find an article by Goodwin and Goodwin (1984) most worthwhile reading.

Advantages and Disadvantages of Fine Needle Aspiration

2

Fine needle aspiration of the breast is a simple, inexpensive, innocuous, accurate, and quick diagnostic method that has many advantages for the patient, the surgeon, the hospital, and the pathologist. The disadvantages are negligible.

ADVANTAGES FOR THE PATIENT

1. It is psychologically more acceptable than a biopsy because it is a simple office procedure that causes little discomfort and does not leave a scar.
2. If a diagnosis of carcinoma is made on aspiration, the patient can be better prepared emotionally for surgery.
3. It helps to reduce hospital costs for patients with carcinoma. When we make a diagnosis of carcinoma on the aspirated material, the surgeon can save time (and money for the patient) by proceeding to perform a mastectomy without excisional biopsy. This will save about 45 minutes in the operating room and may obviate the need for a frozen section or a two-stage mastectomy. "Staging" and/or "metastatic work-up" need be performed only in those cases of carcinoma diagnosed by aspiration cytology.
4. Fine needle aspiration is of special value for definitive diagnosis of clinically inoperable mammary cancer prior to radiotherapy, for a suspected thoracic wall recurrence after mastectomy, and for diagnosing a possible "second cancer" in the opposite breast.
5. In spite of frequent visits to their physicians, it has been reported that

the diagnosis of cancer is delayed in pregnant patients. Surgeons avoid excisional biopsies in this group of patients because of hyperpigmented ugly scars, higher incidence of hematomas and infection, and the interference with lactation. Fine needle aspiration can provide a prompt diagnosis and determine which patients need surgery.

6. The technique is innocuous. Trauma is minimal due to the thin needle used. There is no risk of spreading cancer cells with this procedure, and there is no need for a local anesthetic.

7. It is a rapid method of diagnosis. The aspiration procedure takes only a few minutes, and slides can be stained easily in five minutes. Straightforward cases can be interpreted in only a few minutes more.

8. It is relatively inexpensive.

9. If the lesion is benign, the patient is spared unnecessary anxiety. When a cyst is present, the procedure is not only diagnostic but also therapeutic.

10. It would allow the use of neoadjuvant (preoperative) chemotherapy if such treatment modality becomes accepted (Ragaz et al. 1985).

ADVANTAGES FOR THE SURGEON AND/OR INTERNIST

1. Aspiration is a simple office procedure that can be mastered easily. Special attention should be given to preparation of the smears.

2. The equipment needed is inexpensive.

3. Fine needle aspiration is helpful in patients with masses that the surgeon decides to "follow," such as in cases when
   a. there has been a long history of fibrocystic mastopathy with multiple surgical excisions.
   b. recurrent lumps are present at the site of a surgical scar.
   c. the surgeon is concerned that an excisional biopsy and the ensuing fibrosis will compromise follow-up mammography.
   d. a pregnant patient presents with a large mass that cannot be excised under local anesthesia.

4. Fine needle aspiration can uncover clinically unsuspected carcinoma—a major benefit of the procedure. We have had several cases in which the mass was believed to be benign based on palpation and mammogram, but aspiration revealed malignant cells. These patients benefited from prompt surgical treatment. Our experience is not unique (Malberger et al. 1981, p. 903).

5. The opposite is also true: not all lesions believed to be cancer prove to be so. We have had cases of subareolar abscess with peau d'orange dermal changes, which may resolve after aspiration and antibiotic therapy.

6. A definite preoperative diagnosis allows the surgeon to schedule cases more appropriately and to decide which can be performed on an ambulatory basis and which require general anesthesia.

7. Time in the operating room is decreased by elimination of the biopsy and frozen section.

ADVANTAGES FOR THE HOSPITAL

1. Scheduling in the operating room is more efficient.
2. Patients are evaluated more economically with consequent savings.

ADVANTAGES FOR THE PATHOLOGIST

1. The pathologist is no longer the "invisible" member of the medical team.
2. The pathologist functions as a consultant and is reimbursed as such.
3. There is improved quality control in the pathology department. By this we mean that fine needle aspiration is of value in monitoring diagnoses in surgical pathology and vice versa.

DISADVANTAGES OF FINE NEEDLE ASPIRATION: REAL AND THEORETICAL

1. The method's principal drawback is the false negative diagnosis related to aspiration failures: (a) highly fibrotic cancers from which malignant cells may be difficult to obtain, (b) small lesions (less than 1 cm) that constitute elusive targets, or (c) the nonpalpable mammographically detected lesions. The first two difficulties are lessened as the aspirator develops greater skill and technical expertise.
2. The false positive diagnosis is an enormous source of concern, particularly at institutions like ours where mastectomies are performed without frozen sections and are based on the cytologic diagnosis. I cannot overemphasize the importance of good judgment, a conservative approach to diagnosis, and good communications among pathologists and surgeons to eliminate this problem. In the near future, with the widespread use of lumpectomy, this problem will lose relevance (Fisher 1985). Because no diagnostic method can claim 100% accuracy, we have to realize that false positives happen in any large series (see Marasà and Tomasino 1982, Table III) and most have not led to mastectomy.
3. Learning how to obtain adequate material takes time. Practice makes perfect.
4. Specialized training is essential for the interpretation.
5. There may be some concern on the part of the surgeon about monetary loss. The surgeon is paid more for an excisional biopsy than for a simple office procedure such as fine needle aspiration.
6. Because of limited material (usually two to four smears), no tissue is available for histologic examination or for the analysis of estrogen receptors. However, these objections are no longer valid because estrogen (Poulsen et al. 1979; Lindgren et al. 1980; Curtin et al. 1982; Gunduz et al. 1983) and progesterone (Merle et al. 1985) receptors can be determined on fine needle aspiration smears. Cytologic criteria have been developed to allow a diagnosis of the types of adenocarcinoma with a high degree of accuracy.

COMPLICATIONS

The only complications we have had in our series have been minor bruises and occasional hematomas. Mastitis and/or pneumothorax have been reported occasionally (Abele et al. 1983, p. 861). We are aware that pneumothorax also can occur when aspirating axillary and supraclavicular lymph nodes. So far, we have not caused any. Although this is a simple technique, one should keep in mind that any procedure carelessly performed can be hazardous.

NEEDLE BIOPSIES

This technique is more complicated because it is a surgical procedure that requires anesthesia and asepsis (Foster 1982). With the cutting needle, a tissue "core" is obtained and then processed in the same manner as other tissues. Advantages are:

1. A segment of tissue is obtained which allows the traditional pathologist to feel more comfortable with the interpretation.
2. Multiple sections and stains can be performed easily.

The disadvantages of the technique include:

1. Limited sampling.
2. Patients experience more pain than with fine needle aspiration.
3. Small lesions are missed more easily than with fine needle aspiration.
4. More complications and more trauma occur than with fine needle aspiration. Roberts et al. (1975, Table 2) reported that 33% of their cases experienced significant bleeding.
5. A pressure dressing needs to be applied for 24 hours.

These specimens obtained by needle biopsy also cause some problems for the pathologist:

1. They are very small.
2. Their gross features are difficult to evaluate.
3. Crush artifacts are frequent.
4. Diagnosis requires at least 18 to 24 hours.

There is a need for accurate preoperative diagnosis of breast masses. We concur with Coates et al. (1977, p. 78) that "it is not justifiable to plan definitive therapy on clinical evidence alone." The use of Tru-cut needle biopsies is one step toward satisfying that need (Elston et al. 1978; Raff 1982). At our institution fewer than ten Tru-cut biopsies have been performed. That need is being fulfilled by fine needle aspirations. Others have stated similar preferences (Shabot et al. 1982; Lever et al. 1985, p. 1).

Questions Asked Most Frequently

3

WHY DIFF-QUIK?

In 1976, when I became interested in fine needle aspirations, I used the Papanicolaou stain; then I went to Sweden and discovered that all their material was air-dried and stained with May-Grünwald Giemsa. Initially I resented this because it was alien to me, but that was the only material available. Also, many other Europeans, in addition to the Swedish cytologists, use hematologic stains for this purpose. Thus, I said to myself, "all of Europe cannot be wrong." After overcoming my initial resistance, I found it simpler to diagnose this material.

When we started using the May-Grünwald Giemsa stain, we found it cumbersome to prepare and the staining quality variable. Some smears would stain beautifully; others were not fully satisfactory. Then we came across Diff-Quik, which has solved the problem of stain preparation and is also reliable and rapid. Our only objection through the years has been the constant price increases, so we are trying to find some substitutes.

It is part of the natural process for smears to dry at the edges first. Thin smears, in particular, dry almost immediately. Pathologists and cytotechnologists are aware of this and thus remove the lid of a Coplin jar containing 95% ethanol and drop the smears very promptly in the fixative. However, it is hard to convince surgeons and their assistants about the "air-drying" artifacts caused by delayed fixation. When examining submitted smears (whether alcohol-fixed or spray-fixed) stained with Papanicolaou's method this becomes a constant source of aggravation and, worse, a cause of errors. Wilson and Ehrmann (1978, p. 475) reported, "Our false positive and suspicious readings resulted chiefly from misinterpretation of drying artifacts, reactive or degenerative atypia of cyst

8

wall epithelium, and foreign body reactions." However, if you use hematologic stains you do not need to worry about fixing the material promptly.

Another disadvantage of the alcohol fixation for subsequent Papanicolaou stain is cell loss, which increases the number of false negative aspirates (Chu and Hoye 1973, p. 416).

The diagnostic criteria for material stained with Diff-Quik differ from the diagnostic criteria for material stained with Papanicolaou's technique. We believe that it is much easier and faster to make a diagnosis on hematologically stained smears which simplify the diagnostic criteria. For example, ductal adenocarcinomas are diagnosed at low magnification ($\times 40$) based on "tumor cellularity" and pattern recognition. The nuclear pleomorphism required to confirm the diagnosis is easily observed at medium ($\times 100$) or high magnification ($\times 400$), a factor surgical pathologists will find more appealing. One does not have to spend as much time scrutinizing the nuclei to find or observe the minute details of the chromatin distribution. Cytoplasmic detail and granules are more evident; fibrous connective tissue is readily apparent as is mucus and any other material present in the smears (see Tables 3.1 and 3.2).

Table 3.1
Advantages of Diff-Quik versus Papanicolaou stain

Diff-Quik	*Papanicolaou*
Smears are air-dried. This is technically easier for surgeons and internists who perform the aspirations.	Smears need immediate fixation in 95% ethanol. This requires a special effort to obtain good results.
No cell loss.	Cell loss (you see the material floating off when immersing the slide in alcohol).
Staining time is very short, less than two minutes.	Staining time is at least ten minutes.
Only three staining dishes required.	A minimum of 16 dishes required.
Staining technique easy to master.	More difficult to set up stains. Technical help needed to stain smears.
Smears can be examined wet, without coverslipping, to ensure adequacy of specimen.	Smears have to be coverslipped.
Blood in the background does not interfere with the staining of epithelial cells.	Blood in the background obscures cellular detail.
Cells are larger and more obvious.	Cells shrink due to the alcohol-fixation and alcohol rinses.
Diagnostic criteria are much simpler.	Diagnostic criteria require closer cellular scrutiny under higher magnification.
Cytoplasmic granules, inclusions, connective tissue, and secretions are easier to visualize.	Not evident.

Table 3.2
Disadvantages of Diff-Quik versus Papanicolaou stain

Diff-Quik	Papanicolaou
Pathologist and cytotechnologist need to acquire familiarity with the stain.	Pathologist and cytotechnologist are very familiar with the stain.
Thick smears are difficult to stain adequately.	Nuclear detail can still be appreciated in thick smears.
Squamous cells are somewhat difficult to identify.	Squamous cells are easily recognized.

Most pathologists and cytotechnologists were trained to stain cytologic smears with Papanicolaou's stain and are not inclined to use anything else. Please reconsider. Try the hematologic stains and give them a fair chance. You will profit from it in the long run.

Throughout this monograph all the photographs (unless otherwise specified) and our diagnostic criteria apply specifically to smears stained with Diff-Quik.

Recent books on fine needle aspiration will provide the reader with several choices. Some authors (Linsk and Franzen 1983, pp. 108–135; Schöndorf 1978) are partial to hematologic stains; some (Kline 1981, pp. 118–171; Koss et al. 1984, pp. 56–101) prefer Papanicolaou's stain; and others (Feldman and Covell 1985, pp. 49–115; Frable 1983, pp. 21–68) use both types of stains.

HOW DID WE GET STARTED?

Every time I give a lecture or workshop, some pathologists will ask me how I began and how I convinced the surgeons (in particular) to send me patients for aspirations. They tell me about the frustrations they face in getting started and, alas, it is all so familiar. If you are facing these problems you might benefit from reading what follows. If you have overcome these problems, skip these next paragraphs.

In 1976 after reading several articles on fine needle aspiration, I became enthusiastic about it. I shared this with two surgeons who began aspirating their patients and sending us the smears for interpretation. At this point I realized I should obtain some formal training. My initial steps were taken under the guidance of Dr. Kersti Hedberg, a pathologist at Sahlgrenska Sjukhuset in Göteborg, Sweden. Also, I spent a very worthwhile week at the Karolinska Sjukhuset in Stockholm. When I returned home, I did not miss a chance to let my colleagues know that I was available at any time to perform fine needle aspirations on their patients. Several surgeons allowed me to come to their offices to perform fine needle aspirations. An hour later we would call them with a report. Then the word spread that I was "the only pathologist who made house calls." As the number of aspirations gradually increased, I stopped making "house calls." I explained that I could serve them better if they would send the patients to our laboratory.

My first aspiration room was my office and for about one year I performed aspirations on patients while they sat in a chair. For lesions in the lower quadrants of the breast, the patients had to stand or I had to kneel. My turning point was having a physician's wife faint in my office during the performance of a fine needle aspiration of her thyroid. I believe this helped me obtain an aspiration room and an examining table.

We did not charge for performing the procedure until 1979. A year later, as the number of cases increased, we found it disruptive to our general diagnostic service and teaching responsibilities to have patients drop by the office for fine needle aspirations. Thus, we began an appointment schedule but still allowed the maximum possible flexibility for "walk-ins." The service kept growing, and it became difficult for me to see patients every working day. In 1980 we began a training program; with the help of my first fellow, we saw more patients. In 1982 we doubled our charges but the demand continued. Thus, our staff has grown. The one-year fellowship has been expanded to two years, and I also have trained a full-time staff pathologist to perform fine needle aspirations. An interesting program for staged implementation of fine needle aspiration has been reported by Abele et al. (1983).

Summary

Approach the surgeon who is your closest friend or the one who calls you most frequently for frozen sections.
Do not charge for the procedure.
Go out of your way to perform an aspiration (make "house calls").
Provide reports within the hour.
Obtain adequate training for performing the aspiration and reading the smears.

THE PATIENT AND INFORMED CONSENT

To *inform* means to impart knowledge or information, to supply with knowledge. To *consent* is to permit, approve, or agree; to comply or yield; to give permission or approval of what is done or proposed by another; it is agreement, compliance, acquiescence.

I believe every patient on whom we perform a fine needle aspiration is informed adequately by both the referring physician and by ourselves. The patient is also agreeable to having the procedure performed, not only by coming to our laboratory, but also by collaborating with us in taking the sample. However, we do not ask any patient to sign a formal agreement, and hence we do not have any documentation. I believe that informed consent is a process and not merely a signature on a piece of paper.

THE ASPIRATION TEAM IN THE PATHOLOGY DEPARTMENT

I cannot overemphasize that fine needle aspiration requires *teamwork*. The members of that team are secretaries, cytotechnologists, and pathologists (residents, fellows, and staff). All will have to be instructed in managing these patients. Most of the patients with whom they will work are afraid of cancer or believe that they have cancer. Some will say so in an explicit way, others will show it as anxiety and/or by being difficult or irritable.

The Secretary

The secretary is the first individual to meet the patients, to arrange for appointments, and to give them instructions on how to reach the laboratory. Often the same instructions will have to be repeated several times to the same patient or during the course of a day to many patients. Remember that this can be trying. Each secretary should understand the technique and what it involves. Thus the secretary can help answer the patients' questions.

We have given our secretaries the following advice: When scheduling, try to accommodate patients to the best of your ability. It is better to obtain all the pertinent information (insurance data, referring physician, *etc.*) during a telephone conversation rather than to wait until the patient arrives to have the procedure performed. Some patients are apprehensive and seem to get annoyed easily if they are questioned at that time. Remember that a neat and well-organized office inspires a sense of confidence. Attractive posters on the walls are a distraction that is appreciated by the patients and make for a more pleasant experience than had been anticipated. Most of all the secretary must be patient and helpful.

The Cytotechnologist

Working with patients is not a skill acquired during the technologist's training, so the pathologist will have to provide this instruction. In addition, the technologist must learn to answer the many questions asked by anxious patients.

Our cytotechnologists have the following suggestions: After greeting the patient, it is important to take a few moments to explain the procedure. Some patients are not sure of what is going to happen, or if they are, restating it or discussing it seems to relieve some anxiety. It is also helpful to be able to converse with the patients or to make small talk to calm them and put them at ease.

The cytotechnologists also help the patients get undressed before calling the pathologist. They assist with the procedure and help with smear preparation. They stain the smears and do the the initial screening before coverslipping them. Remember, a coverslip is more expensive than the regular glass slide. If some of the smears show only blood, the cytotechnologist will leave them on the tray without coverslipping. On reviewing the case later, the pathologist can determine that indeed those smears are worthless and can be discarded.

The Pathologist

The pathologist must develop or reacquire palpatory ability. Performing fine needle aspirations demonstrates how your hands are an extension of your intellect. Discipline, dedication, and much work are needed. Do not forget that when you deal with patients you have to be compassionate (Vickery 1983). Remember, you must learn the "how-to," but you also have to have good clinical judgment. Although the technique seems simple, it must be learned, and it takes time to develop expertise. Those surgical pathologists trained in the conventional manner will have to acquire cytologic expertise. The diagnosis of a smear is only as good as the person reading it.

You have to know yourself. If you are a sprinter rather than a long distance runner, then fine needle aspiration is not for you. The most important characteristic required in a pathologist performing fine needle aspirations is persistence. So many roadblocks exist that if you do not persevere the service will never flourish. You will be facing the skepticism of surgeons, clinicians, and also of some fellow pathologists. Today with interventional radiology growing in many hospitals, you can count on help from the radiologists.

Cytotechnologists and pathologists seeing patients should take a course in cardiopulmonary resuscitation. Very seldom will you need this information but if a patient faints, the aspiration team can then manage the episode with confidence.

It is the policy of our department that no patient is addressed by her or his first name. It is more professional and respectful to address a patient by her surname (King 1985).

THE ASPIRATION ROOM

An appropriate setting for performing fine needle aspirations should be provided. This includes a waiting area (as in any other physician's office) and an examining room or aspiration room that is comfortable and allows privacy. Remember that when patients are undressed and wearing only a paper gown, the temperature of the room should not be cold.

In our experience, having an aspiration room has only advantages. The pathologist can perform many more aspirations than when journeying to different nursing stations or offices to perform the procedure. The smears can be checked immediately, and the patient can be reaspirated until diagnostic material is obtained. It makes better use of professional time and hence is more economical. We perform aspirations in a patient's room only if the patient is nonambulatory.

In our cytopathology laboratory we have a room that is only used for performing and processing aspirates. The room is divided into two sections. In front is the patient area, and behind a partition is the staining and processing area. In the patient area we have an examining table, a small table with the materials required for the aspiration, two chairs, and a countertop that serves as a desk. There is also a place to hang the patients' clothes. The cytotechnologist on duty will explain the procedure to the patient, help the patient undress, supply a disposable paper gown, and ask the patient to sit on the examining table. Then the pathologist will be called into the room.

THE CRUX OF THE MATTER

What should be aspirated? Any palpable lesion of the breast, whether it is a discrete nodule or mass, or an ill-defined "thickening," should be aspirated (Fig. 3.1).

When should it be aspirated? It should be aspirated as soon as the patient or her physician discovers it. We strongly object to the attitude of "let's wait and see what happens," when dealing with a mass. The key to successful management of patients lies in an early diagnosis. With fine needle aspiration you have the means to solve the diagnostic problem if you choose to do so.

Why do an aspiration? It should be done because the appropriate management of the lesion will depend to a large extent on the diagnosis provided by the aspiration. Fine needle aspiration is such a simple procedure that it can be scheduled almost immediately. Provisions should be made to accept walk-in patients. It should be easier to get an appointment for an aspiration than for a mammogram.

Figure 3.1.
Management of palpable masses.

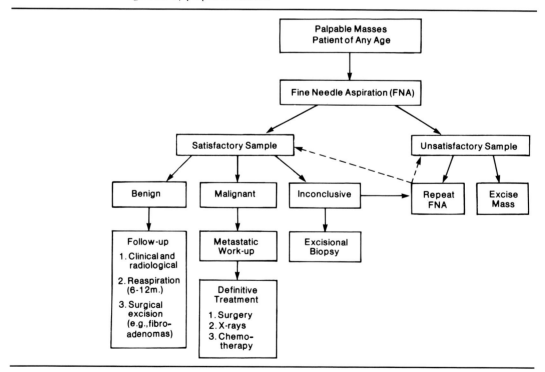

Who should do it? It is preferable that the aspiration be performed by the pathologist. The accuracy rate of diagnoses is higher when the pathologist performs the aspiration. The advantages and disadvantages of nonpathologists performing aspirations have been discussed previously (Oertel 1982). However, some internists and many surgeons will continue performing fine needle aspirations and submitting material to pathologists.

Where should it be aspirated? It is preferable that aspirations take place in the cytopathology service, where an "aspiration room" should be available. As this is an outpatient procedure, any physician's office is suitable.

Now, let me pose this question to you: *Will you do it?* I believe every pathologist should be prepared to perform and interpret fine needle aspirations because this is the pathology of the future. The new methods of reimbursement are going to "encourage" us to do it, and they will not allow pathologists to seek refuge behind the "paraffin curtain." A pathologist proficient in performing the aspirates will be able to provide sound advice to colleagues. Everybody benefits. Remember, you cannot give what you do not have. You cannot train other physicians to perform the procedure if you do not know how to do it yourself. Nor can you offer advice and help solve problems unless you have had personal experience.

Fine Needle Aspiration Technique

4

Although we have covered this subject in two previous publications (Oertel 1982; Oertel and Galblum 1983), for the sake of completeness it is reviewed briefly here. We must remember that the ultimate goal is an accurate and prompt diagnosis and that whatever we do must contribute to this goal.

We must (1) avoid loss of cells; (2) avoid distortion of the cells; (3) use inexpensive stains without compromising quality; (4) adopt a simple staining method.

The technique will be successful if an adequate sample is obtained, handled, and processed in the best possible way. You may obtain an excellent sample, but if it is not smeared correctly it will be worthless. The same applies to the staining. As in surgical pathology, much depends on the quality of the material you are going to examine. Attention to detail is indispensable.

WHAT IS NEEDED TO PERFORM AN ASPIRATION?

The equipment required is simple and inexpensive and is described below.

Syringe Holder (or Handle)

We consider the syringe holder to be an indispensable item (Fig. 4.1). It allows the physician to fix or secure the lesion with one hand, making it an easy target,

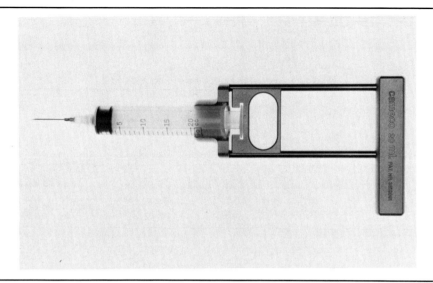

Figure 4.1.
Equipment used for fine needle aspiration of the breast.

and also allows application of suction, which guarantees a more generous sample. There are three types of syringe handles available on the market:

Cameco Syringe Pistol
Precision Dynamics Corporation
3031 Thornton Avenue
Burbank, California 91504

Aspir Gun
The Everest Company
7 Sherman Street
Linden, New Jersey 07036

Reusable Syringe Holder
Medical R H Products
9510 Forest Road
Bethesda, Maryland 20014

Plastic Syringe

We use 20-cc disposable plastic syringes with Luer-Lok tip, available from Becton-Dickinson, Division of Becton Dickinson and Company, Rutherford, New Jersey 07070.

Needles

We recommend disposable needles, 22-gauge, 1.0 inch and 1.5 inches long, with *clear plastic hubs*. These needles are available from Sherwood Medical Industries, Monoject Scientific Division, 1831 Olive, St. Louis, Missouri 63103.

For several years we have been advocating the clear plastic hub, which we find extremely useful. It has two advantages: Because you will not stop the suction until some material appears in the needle hub, there are no "dry taps"; and you will be able to release the suction before any of the specimen goes into the syringe.

Initially, when we perceived that we were not obtaining adequate material with a 22-gauge needle, we would switch to a 21-gauge and, occasionally, to a 20-gauge. Our logic was "the bigger the needle, the more generous the sample." We found this not to be true. The larger the needle, the more blood is aspirated and the greater the likelihood of giving the patient a hematoma. When using a handle, there is no need for a needle larger than a 22-gauge.

Glass Slides

We prefer the Up-Rite microslides with one frosted end, from Richard Allen Medical Industries. Because they are etched UP-RITE (Fig. 4.2), it is not difficult to place the specimen on the same side. When staining and wiping the slide dry, you will not wipe away the sample by accident. Necessary patient identification can be written easily with a pencil on the frosted end.

Some pathologists advocate the use of albuminized slides in order to allow more cells to stick to the slides. Others prefer all frosted slides for the same purpose. In our opinion, both have more drawbacks than benefits. Albumin produces background staining that interferes with the interpretation. All-frosted slides cause artifactual stretching and elongation of cells, evident as marked "spindling" of the cells.

Hemacytometer Cover Glass

This is a thick piece of glass, narrower than the width of the regular glass microslide (Fig. 4.2), which we have been using for years and find very helpful. The hemacytometer cover glass is more satisfactory than using another microslide to make the smears because (1) it causes less crushing and distortion of cells, and (2) it provides a border or edge to the smear where most of the cells will be concentrated; this allows faster screening and diagnosis.

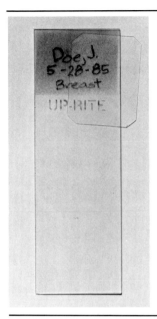

Figure 4.2.
Glass slide and hemacytometer cover glass.

HOW TO PERFORM THE ASPIRATION

After the customary greeting, ask the patient to place a finger on the lump. If the mass is located in the upper quadrants, she may remain seated for the aspiration. The cytotechnologist will raise the back of the table to offer support for the patient's back, making sure to mention that the table will be moving. Most patients are apprehensive and if you are not careful to explain every detail of the procedure, they will overreact and be frightened unnecessarily. If the lump is in the lower aspect of the breast, tell the patient that it will be easier for you to palpate and aspirate while she is lying down.

Before performing the aspiration, ask the patient if she knows what you are going to do. Most of the time the patient will say, "I guess so, but you better explain it to me again." Take this opportunity to discuss the following:

1. The needle used is thinner than that used for venipuncture. Hence the procedure is going to be less painful than drawing blood from a vein.
2. There will be no need for anesthesia. The prick of the needle for the anesthetic would hurt as much as the aspiration. We also believe that the use of anesthetic has two disadvantages: if the nodule is small, any fluid injected will mask the lesion and decrease the chances of hitting it; if the lesion is superficial, the sample will be diluted with the anesthetic fluid. In addition, the anesthetic causes damage to the cells (explosion of the cytoplasm).

3. It is necessary to insert a needle at least twice to obtain enough cells for an adequate diagnosis. I have not yet had a patient refuse a repeat sampling.

Proceed in the following way:

1. Grasp the mass with your nondominant hand between your thumb and forefinger in a position suitable for needling. At other times, it will be easier to push the mass against a rib, holding it between your middle finger and forefinger.
2. Clean the skin with a cotton swab soaked in ethyl alcohol (Fig. 4.3A). Dry the skin with a gauze sponge to avoid the sting caused by residual alcohol when inserting the needle.
3. Introduce the needle through the skin, making sure that the syringe is in "the resting position" (plunger at the "0" cc mark) (Fig. 4.3B).
4. Advance the needle into the mass.
5. Once the needle has entered the lesion, apply suction (pulling the plunger of the syringe to the 20-cc mark) (Fig. 4.3C).
6. Move the needle back and forth (in the same plane) in the mass, maintaining the suction until some material appears in the clear plastic needle hub.
7. *Release the plunger* (Fig. 4.3D).
8. Withdraw the needle.
9. Ask the patient to apply pressure at the site of the aspiration, using the same piece of gauze that you used to dry the skin in Step 2.

Note: *Do not skip Step 7.* It is a common mistake for beginners to withdraw the needle from the mass while still applying suction. This will cause all the aspirated material to flow into the syringe, and you will be left with no sample to smear and will need to repeat the entire procedure using a new syringe and needle.

It has been emphasized in the literature (Zajicek 1974, pp. 4−5; Frable 1984, p. 672) that the needle should be moved widely in the lesion (or redirected while still within the lesion) to obtain a more representative sample. It has been my experience that this only succeeds in giving the patient a hematoma and diluting the sample with blood. Better results are obtained by just moving the needle back and forth along the same axis (Fig. 4.4). The adjacent portions of the lesion are similarly sampled (Steps 1−9) using another needle and syringe. The number of needles used will depend on the lesion's size.

Do not insert the needle through the areola when a subareolar lesion is present. It is too painful. Use a 1-1/2−inch needle, even if the lesion is superficial, and approach it laterally or from behind through the parenchyma of the breast.

Mammograms should not be done immediately after fine needle aspiration because they might be misinterpreted and lead to false positive diagnosis. At least two weeks should elapse before a mammogram is performed (Sickles et al. 1983, pp. 396−397).

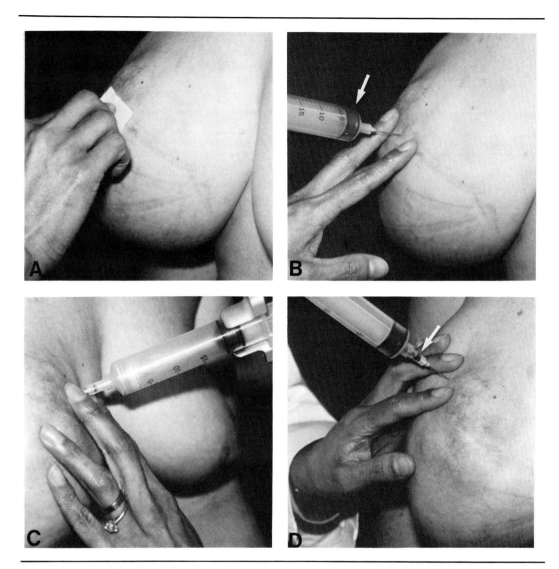

Figure 4.3.
Performance of fine needle aspiration. A. Cleanse the skin with alcohol-soaked cotton swab. B. Insert the needle into the lesion. Notice that the syringe plunger is at the "O cc" mark (arrow). C. Apply suction. Notice that the syringe plunger is at the "20cc" mark. D. Aspirated material is visible in the clear plastic needle hub (arrow); suction is no longer applied because we are about to withdraw the needle.

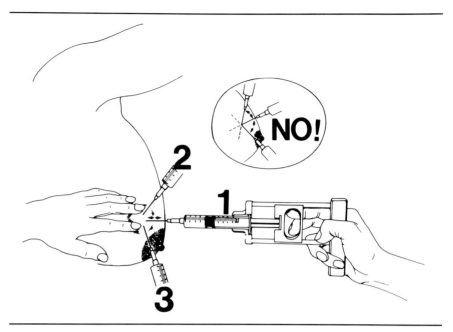

Figure 4.4.
Diagram illustrating three different aspirations of the same mass (center, top, *and* bottom).

PREPARATION OF THE SMEARS

The aspirated material tends to clot quickly, and there should be no delay in preparing the smears.

1. Detach the needle from the syringe (Fig. 4.5A).
2. Fill the syringe with air (Fig. 4.5B).
3. Reattach the needle to the syringe.
4. Place the bevel of the needle against the glass slide and squirt the contents of the needle onto the slide (one drop on each slide) (Fig. 4.5C).
5. Using a hemacytometer cover glass, smear the cellular material as if it were a blood smear (Figs. 4.5D–F).
6. Let smears air-dry.
7. The air-dried smears are then ready for staining and interpretation.

Figure 4.5.
Preparation of the smears. A. Detach the needle from the syringe. B. Fill the syringe with air. C. Place a drop of the aspirated material on each slide. D. Place the hemacytometer cover glass in front of the drop. E. Move the cover glass back to touch the drop of aspirated material and wait for it to spread along the edge of the hemacytometer cover glass. F. Move the cover glass forward.

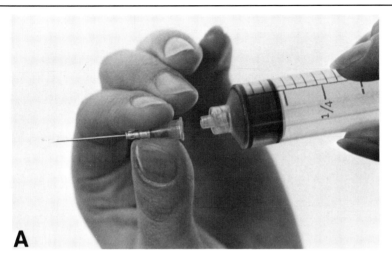

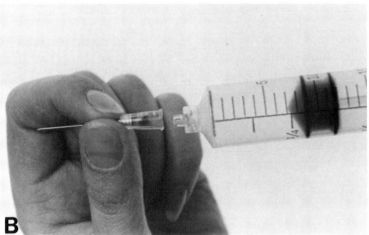

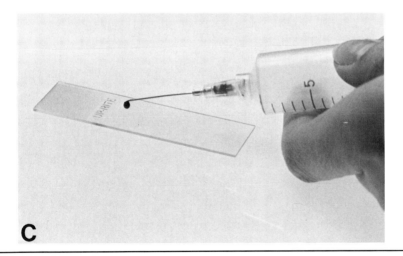

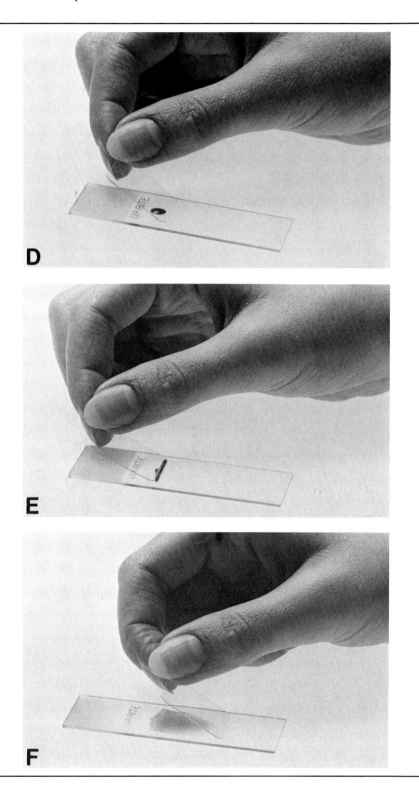

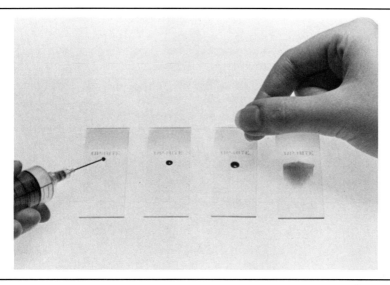

Figure 4.6.
While the pathologist empties the contents of the needle hub onto the glass slides, the cytotechnologist prepares the smears.

Repeat Steps 1 through 4 as many times as needed to empty the material present in the needle hub. Usually three or four smears are prepared from the contents of each needle using the same hemacytometer cover glass (Fig. 4.6). Forcing air through the needle several times, until the hub appears empty, allows recovery of all the material. We have tried rinsing the needles and then preparing Millipore filters or Cytospin smears but found practically nothing left to examine.

When the drop of the material placed on the glass slide appears thick or semisolid, pick up the glass slide (by the frosted end) with your left hand, and hold the hemacytometer cover glass with your right hand, apply pressure, and spread the drop as shown in Figures 4.7A–C.

The soiled hemacytometer cover glasses are placed in a plastic container of soapy water and later are rinsed, dried, and made ready for reuse.

STAINING OF THE SMEARS

We stain the smears with Diff-Quik, manufactured by Dade Diagnostics, Inc., Aguada, Puerto Rico 00602, and distributed by Scientific Products. This staining procedure is simple, fast, and consistently provides good results. We do not use Papanicolaou's stain for breast aspirates anymore nor do we use filter preparations; they are too expensive and cumbersome. We use only direct smears.

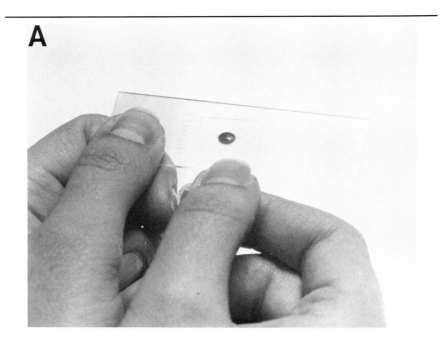

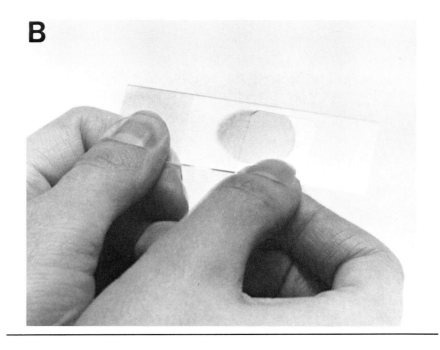

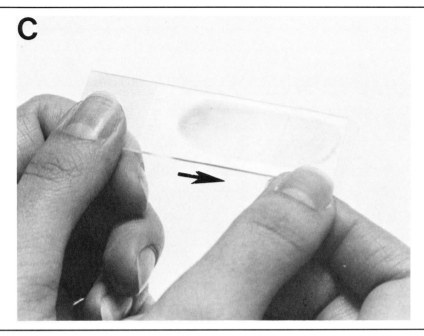

Figure 4.7.
"Crush" method of smearing. A. Hold the glass slide with your left hand and the hemacytometer cover glass with your right hand, on top of the aspirated material. B. Press the hemacytometer cover glass with your right thumb against the aspirate. C. Move horizontally toward the opposite end of the slide.

The first smear from each aspirate is stained immediately, while the patient is still in the aspiration room. This has the following advantages:

1. The patient does not leave the room until a satisfactory specimen is obtained. Patients are most cooperative once you explain that this will avoid their having to return for reaspiration.
2. When dealing with an abscess or a granulomatous process, subsequent aspirates can be sent to the microbiology laboratory for culture.
3. Additional aspirates from unusual cases can be processed for electron microscopy or immunocytochemistry.
4. Checking one smear after each aspiration allows you to reassure the patient that you will not insert more needles than necessary.
5. This approach reduces the number of unsatisfactory specimens and false negative and "suspicious" diagnoses.

We use a small electric hairdryer to dry the smears quickly. Dip the smear in the fixative solution five or six times. Blot the slide on a paper towel and dip six or seven times in solution #1 (cytoplasmic stain). Blot the slide again before dipping in solution #2. Depending upon the age of this solution, three to five, or more, immersions will be required. If the solution is new, it is preferable to rinse the slide in tap water after three dips and then to check the nuclear stain under the microscope. If the nuclei are too pale, you can go back and dip the slide several more times in solution #2. Remember that it is much easier to correct understaining than overstaining. After rinsing in tap water, blot the slide. The remaining slides can be stained in batches of 25 or 50, depending on the size of your staining rack and containers.

A word of caution: You can use a hairdryer or any heat source to dry the smears before staining. Once the smears have been *stained*, they should be *air-dried at room temperature ONLY*. Do not use a hairdryer, a slide warmer, or any source of heat to dry *stained* smears. In our experience, this ruins the quality of the stain and makes the colors appear dull. After the smears have dried at room temperature, place them in xylene and then coverslip with any available mounting medium ; or it may be easier to directly coverslip the smears without soaking them in xylene. Do *not* use any alcohol because it decolorizes the smears. Once the smears have been coverslipped, they can be dried *gently* on a slide warmer.

Always keep the staining solutions closed when not in use, particularly solution #2; otherwise a film forms on it which precipitates on the smears (see Figs. 7.6 and 7.7). When staining in batches, the smears may be left in the fixative for any length of time, even overnight. You can also leave the smears in solution #1 for several hours without danger of overstaining. The only critical step is the one involving solution #2.

HOW TO LEARN TO PERFORM THE PROCEDURE

The pathologist must become familiar with the syringe handle and the syringe. In our service we begin training residents and fellows by using an apple. This has many advantages. It is less messy than practicing with tissue specimens, and it provides them with a simulation of the grittiness felt when aspirating a mammary carcinoma. The next step, which I consider invaluable, is to observe an experienced pathologist perform the procedure on several patients. Then a role reversal should occur; the experienced pathologist watches the novice perform the procedure. After the patient has departed, the pathologist can advise improvements in the technique. I cannot overemphasize the advantages of having an experienced teacher.

How to Succeed at Fine Needle Aspiration 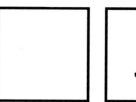 5

Success in fine needle aspiration is most likely if the pathologist performs the procedure. In the beginning you will encounter considerable resistance from clinicians and surgeons who are not accustomed to referring patients to a pathologist. But once they realize the economy of time and money of such referral and the increase in diagnostic accuracy, your problems will be solved. I would advise you to approach first those surgeons with whom you most frequently work in the operating room. If they trust your frozen section diagnoses, they will trust you with their patients.

Fine needle aspiration will work if you communicate with the referring physician, keep the interests of the patients in mind, and enlist their cooperation during the procedures. Likewise, you must use your clinical acumen and correlate it with the microscopic findings. If you believe that fine needle aspiration is merely a matter of inserting a needle and withdrawing a few cells from a lump, the procedure will not work. It is necessary for pathologists to understand that they have to spend time with the patients, examine them carefully, and develop a high index of suspicion for any abnormalities in the breasts. There is a trade-off: either you spend your time looking at poor material submitted by surgeons, internists, and general practitioners, or you spend your time with the patient and obtain the best possible samples.

Self-examination of the breasts is an effective means of detecting breast cancer, but most American women continue to ignore its importance. Try to become another source of information on self-examination. In our office we keep brochures from the American Cancer Society on this technique. We also teach patients how to perform the self-examination and encourage them to do it monthly on "the day the telephone bill comes" (Sullivan 1985).

WHAT IS AN ADEQUATE SAMPLE?

This is a difficult question to answer. It is similar to the pathology resident who asks, "How many sections should I take from a surgical specimen?" There are so many variables involved that I can offer only general guidelines.

1. If a needle can enter a lesion, something can be aspirated. Even with fibrotic lesions, some material can be obtained, whether it is collagenous fibers or a few connective tissue cells. There is no acceptable excuse for a blank smear or for a dry tap. If one uses a clear hub needle, the suction should be continued, and the needle should be moved back and forth in the lesion until some material enters the clear hub.
2. When a scirrhous carcinoma is suspected but no cells are seen on the smear, the next aspiration should be more peripheral. Once you feel the grittiness of the lesion with the needle, do not go any deeper; on the contrary, try to withdraw somewhat to the softer edge and aspirate the malignant cells infiltrating the fat.
3. In cases of fibrous mastopathy, the consistency of the lesion is quite rubbery, and you will have trouble moving the needle (it bends). These aspirations tend to be very scant. The same advice applies: do not release the suction until you see some material in the needle hub.
4. If you palpate a rather soft, discrete lesion that on aspiration offers no resistance to the needle, and all that is obtained after multiple aspirates is abundant adipose tissue, consider this an adequate sample of a lipoma, in which case you may not see any ductal epithelial cells.
5. Obtain enough material to explain the nature of the palpable mass. For example, a discrete mass with a rubbery consistency on needling found in a young woman is most likely a fibroadenoma. Can you make that diagnosis from the smears?
6. When the woman is postmenopausal or elderly, every palpable breast mass should be considered malignant until proven otherwise. If you are not aspirating malignant cells, persist within reason, but avoid hurting the patient, until you obtain a diagnostic sample. Remember the ancient dictum "first do no harm."
7. Try to put yourself in the patient's place. If it were a lesion in your breast, would you think it had been sampled appropriately?
8. Aspirate as many times as the patient will allow you to do so. Rarely will you have "too much" material.

Diagnostic accuracy depends on the adequacy of the sample. Evaluate the specimen based on your clinical appraisal of the lesion and by continually asking yourself, "Have I done my best?"

Always be concerned about the possibility of breast cancer. Every patient who comes for a breast aspirate should have her axillae and supraclavicular regions examined. If any nodules are palpable, aspirate them.

UNSATISFACTORY SPECIMENS

We diagnose the following as unsatisfactory or inadequate specimens: (1) smears that show only blood; (2) smears from young women in which only adipose tissue is observed but no ductal epithelial cells (with the exception of lipomas mentioned above); and (3) acellular proteinaceous material.

The concept of unsatisfactory or insufficient specimens is not shared by some (Kern 1979, p. 1126). We would like to reiterate our opinion and that of others (Strawbridge et al. 1981, p. 5; Bell et al. 1983, p. 1188), that an unsatisfactory smear is inadequate for cytologic diagnosis.

When the pathologist performs the aspiration, failure will occur in about 1% of cases. In such instances we do not charge for performing the procedure or reading the smears. If we request a repeat sample and this is performed within three months, we do not charge either. When surgeons and internists submit slides and we have trouble interpreting them because of the material's poor quality (too few cells, or poor smearing technique, *etc.*), we ask the referring physician to send the patient to our office for reaspiration, without an additional charge (Santos 1983). Please note, however, that we do charge the patient if a surgeon reaspirates without our request.

Breast masses have been the most commonly aspirated lesions in our institution. Recently, however, thyroid nodules (Fig. 1.2) have become more numerous.

REASONS FOR UNSATISFACTORY SPECIMENS

The leading cause of unsatisfactory specimens is the physician (see Table 18.4) with defective technique.

1. Not using the handle. Try pulling the plunger of a 20-cc syringe with one hand. Can you apply adequate suction with one hand? To apply adequate suction, you have to release the mass and use both hands (one to hold the syringe, the other to pull the plunger); this will cause you to miss the target and aspirate adjacent tissues but not the lesion.
2. Use of local anesthetic that may mask the lesion, dilute the specimen, and distort or explode the cells.
3. Improper position of the patient and/or poor localization of the lesion; the inexperienced operator performs the procedure immediately rather than after having taken the time needed to place the patient in optimal position.
4. Too vigorous and sudden suction, which creates bleeding.
5. Too big a needle. In theory, a larger bore needle would be expected to yield more rather than fewer cells. In practice, only more blood is obtained, rather than more epithelial cells.
6. Moving the needle in a fanlike fashion (rather than maintaining it in the same direction), which causes bleeding (Fig. 4.4).
7. Pumping the plunger, rather than gently and steadily applying suction.

Once an adequate degree of suction has been reached, move the needle back and forth in the mass.

8. Dry taps, due to insufficient suction, which are unknown to the operator unless clear plastic hub needles are used.

9. Forgetting to release suction before withdrawing the needle from the breast.

10. If physicians other than pathologists are performing the aspirations, they have no way of checking the sample to make sure the specimen is adequate by quickly staining one smear. They also typically fail to reaspirate the lesion at least once more.

11. Overconfidence. The technique is deceptively simple. It is a chain of simple steps that have to be followed meticulously with careful attention to each detail.

12. Very small tumors and/or very fibrous tumors. The small tumors are a difficult target and the needle may go through them. Sclerotic lesions do not yield many cells.

13. Less frequently, unsatisfactory specimens will be due to poor smearing technique.

WHY IS A PARTICULAR ASPIRATION PERFORMED?

Fine needle aspiration should be utilized to answer specific questions (Fig. 3.1):

Is the Mass Solid or Cystic?

Even when you suspect that a cyst is present, use the handle and a 22-gauge needle. You do not need a larger needle to evacuate the fluid, and consequently it will be less painful for the patient. Cysts should be aspirated to relieve the discomfort and to confirm the clinical impression. If the fluid is clear and the lump disappears, no further treatment other than careful follow-up is necessary. As a rule, we immediately reaspirate the region in which the cyst was located (even if there is no residual mass), using a new needle and syringe. When the contents of a cyst are under pressure, the palpable mass may be quite firm. Thus it comes as a surprise to obtain fluid on aspiration.

Although we do not include cysts in our fine needle aspiration series, we advocate needling them. This is one instance in which the procedure is both diagnostic and therapeutic. Also, the patients are extremely grateful once the mass disappears.

Is the Mass Benign or Malignant?

Palpation and physical examination are fairly reliable in making this appraisal, but they are not always accurate. So the physician in the past has traveled two routes: either following the patient and seeing what happened or obtaining a mammogram. During follow-up, the physician watched for a change in the size of the mass (and whether this change correlated with onset of menses) and a change in the character of the mass. One problem is that mammograms are difficult to interpret in younger women with dense fibrous breasts. Another problem is the high rate of false negative diagnosis that "makes mammography an unreliable method to ascertain the nature of a palpable mass" (Newsome and McLelland 1986). And of course, as with any other technique, it also has some false positive diagnoses. Fine needle aspiration can improve the overall accuracy in assessing the lesions. The diagnostic reliability of physical examination, mammography, and fine needle aspiration used in combination seems to be unrivaled (Rimsten et al. 1975; Thomas et al. 1978; Azzarelli et al. 1983; and Dixon et al. 1984).

What Should Be Done Next?

1. Follow-up;
2. Excisional biopsy;
3. Search for metastatic foci if indicated;
4. Mastectomy or lumpectomy;
5. Radiation therapy or chemotherapy; and
6. Proceed with appropriate referral. (For example, a young woman with a family history of breast cancer presented with an axillary mass thought to be a metastatic carcinoma of the breast. On aspiration the lesion was diagnosed as a schwannoma. Needless to say, the patient's anxiety was relieved immediately and a search for metastatic disease was avoided. The general surgeon referred the patient to a neurosurgeon who excised the tumor.)

In summary, learn the technique and become proficient at it, make the commitment to learn to interpret the smears, be available to your colleagues, be kind to patients, train your cytotechnologists, persist, and use good judgment.

Usual Findings in the Aspirates

6

ADIPOSE TISSUE

Adipose tissue is a constant component of the aspirates, sometimes represented by a small fragment consisting of a few adipose cells (with delicate cytoplasmic membranes and small nuclei pushed toward one side), and occasional delicate capillaries (Fig. 6.1). More often you will observe large fragments of tissue that frequently are folded. Sometimes the cytoplasm of the cells will have many small vacuoles, resembling brown fat (Fig. 6.2). In other instances the fragments consist of a mixture of adipose tissue and fibrocollagenous tissue (Figs. 6.3 and 6.4).

NORMAL DUCTAL CELLS

Ductal cells are seen frequently in tightly cohesive, small groups (Fig. 6.5; Color Plate I) and in sheets or monolayers of variable sizes (Figs. 6.6 and 6.7). The nuclei are fairly regular, round to oval, and are about the size of a red blood cell. Nucleoli are seen rarely. The cytoplasm is scanty, often barely visible. In other instances these cells are loosely cohesive (Fig. 6.8A) or may form intercellular lumina or acinar structures (Fig. 6.8B).

34

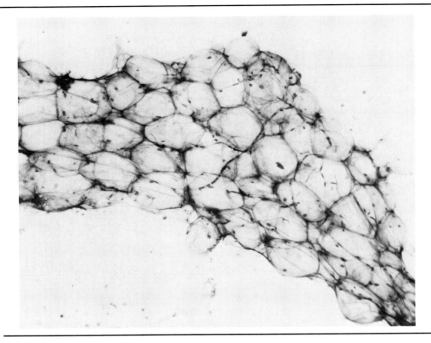

Figure 6.1.
Fragment of adipose tissue (×100).

Figure 6.2.
Adipose tissue with vacuolated cells resembling brown fat (×200).

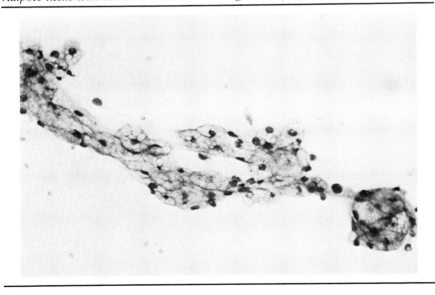

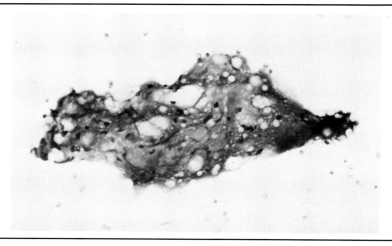

Figure 6.3.
Fragment of fibroadipose tissue with some erythrocytes in the background (×200).

Figure 6.4.
Fibroadipose tissue, same as Figure 6.3 but at higher magnification (×400).

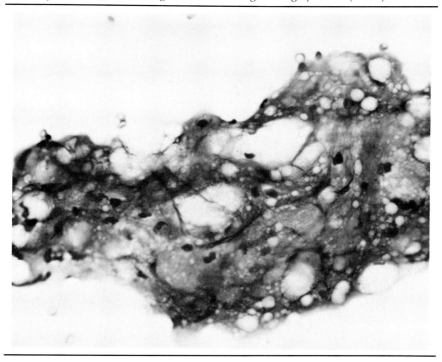

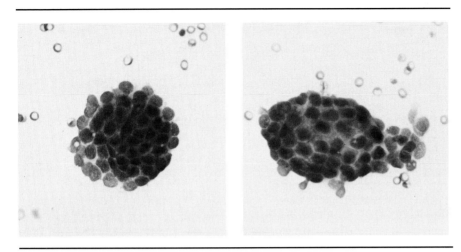

Figure 6.5.
Two small groups of benign ductal epithelial cells (×400).

Figure 6.6.
A sheet of ductal epithelial cells and myoepithelial cells (×200).

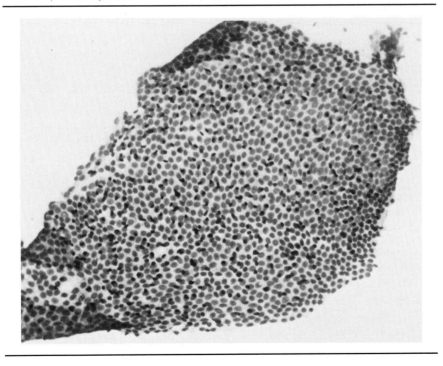

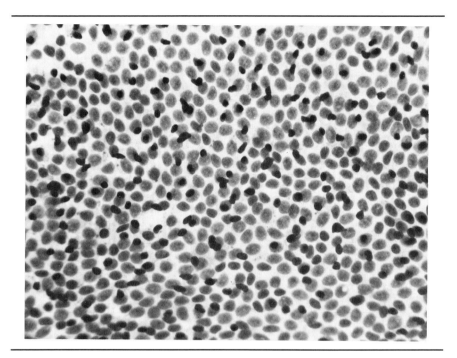

Figure 6.7.
A sheet of ductal epithelial cells and myoepithelial cells (same as in Figure 6.6) (×400).

MYOEPITHELIAL CELLS

In the monolayers of ductal epithelial cells, with their round, regular nuclei, there are occasionally smaller, darker nuclei that sometimes adopt an ovoid shape. These are interpreted as myoepithelial cell nuclei (Figs. 6.6 and 6.7) and are more readily apparent in fibroadenomas.

STRIPPED NUCLEI

Stripped nuclei are ovoid to round, regular nuclei, without cytoplasm, that are scattered throughout the smears. They originate from either fibroblasts or myoepithelial cells and are rather inconspicuous (except in fibroadenomas). They also are referred to as *stripped bipolar nuclei* and *sentinel nuclei* (Fig. 8.36A).

APOCRINE METAPLASTIC CELLS

Apocrine cells are readily recognizable under low magnification (Figs. 6.9A and B). They appear either as large clusters of cells with scalloped borders or as sheets of large polygonal cells. The nuclei are round and larger than those of

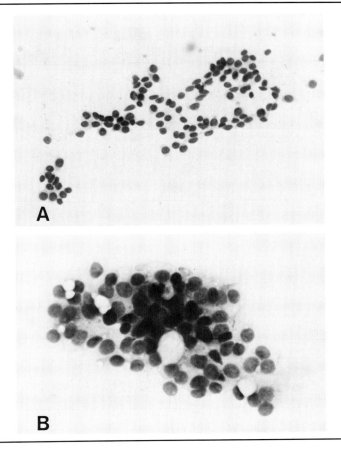

Figure 6.8.
Ductal epithelial cells. A. Loosely cohesive cells (×200). B. Groups of cells containing intercellular lumina (×400).

normal ductal cells (two to three times the size of a red blood cell) and vary in size. The nucleoli are usually conspicuous. The cytoplasm is abundant and has well-demarcated borders (Fig. 6.9C; Color Plate I). Frequently it is dense, gray-pink to pale blue, and contains bluish granules. At other times it is delicate or quite pale and vacuolated (Figs. 6.9D and E). All these variations may be observed in a single cluster of cells.

HISTIOCYTES

These histiocytes are similar to the histiocytes (macrophages or foam cells) found in other organs. They are generally seen either singly or in small loosely cohesive groups. The cytoplasm is pale and has multiple vacuoles that vary in size. Sometimes it contains dark blue granules that vary in size (hemosiderin pigment) (Fig. 6.10). The nuclei are relatively small, round to irregular, and are eccentrically placed. Sometimes the nucleolus is conspicuous.

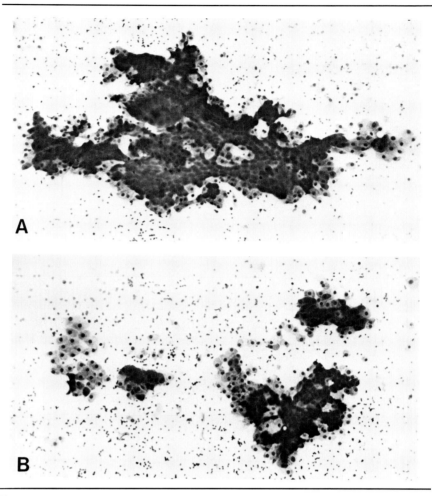

Figure 6.9.
Apocrine metaplastic cells. A. Large irregular groups with dense cytoplasm (×100). B. Smaller groups, one with pale cytoplasm, the others with predominantly dense cytoplasm (×100). C. Note the well-demarcated cellular borders (×400). D. Small group with clearing of cytoplasm, scalloped borders, and degenerated nuclei (×400). E. Larger group with thick cellular borders and clear cytoplasm. An occasional cell has dense cytoplasm (arrow) (×400).

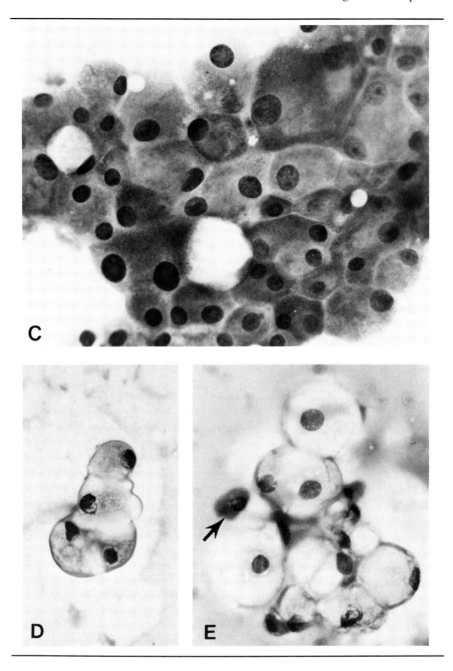

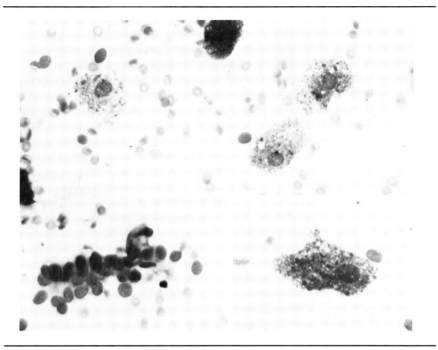

Figure 6.10.
Several histiocytes with hemosiderin granules in the cytoplasm (better appreciated in inset). A clump of benign ductal cells in lower left corner (×400 and inset ×400).

Figure 6.11.
Oleic acid crystals (×400).

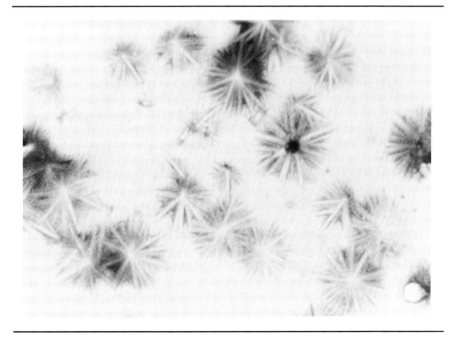

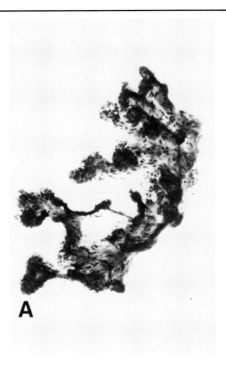

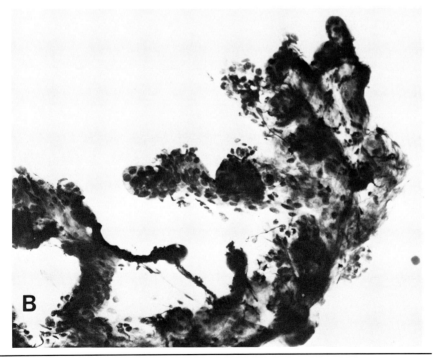

Figure 6.12.
A. *Fragment of breast parenchyma (×100).* B. *Same as* A. *Acini have small regular nuclei. Note connective tissue (×200).*

OLEIC ACID CRYSTALS

Oleic acid crystals are frequently found in aspirates, particularly when there is abundant adipose tissue. These non-birefringent, needle-shaped crystals are seen adjacent to the adipose tissue or in a proteinaceous background. As a rule they are numerous and have the appearance of a sunburst (Fig. 6.11).

BREAST LOBULES

Tissue fragments of the mammary parenchyma have a distinctive appearance at low magnification (Fig. 6.12A) and resemble a branching coral. At higher magnification the epithelial cells that form the acini display regular nuclei. Variable amounts of connective tissue and sometimes blood vessels are present (Fig. 6.12B).

Occasional Findings in the Aspirates

7

SKELETAL MUSCLE

When aspirating the upper outer quadrant, you may sample the pectoralis major, and if the patient has small breasts, when aspirating the lower quadrants, you may obtain some serratus anterior or even intercostal muscle. At low magnification many large, irregular, bluish fragments of tissue are seen (Fig. 7.1A). They appear less cellular (Fig. 7.1B) than the breast lobules (compare with Fig. 6.12). At higher magnification, cross-striations are identified easily, and ovoid to cigar-shaped elongated nuclei are observed (Fig. 7.1C).

SKIN

Skin is easily recognized because the fragments (Fig. 7.2) include a stratum corneum, sometimes a granular layer, a very prominent stratum spinosum, and papillae with connective tissue. Occasionally one will find large clusters of anucleated squamous cells (Fig. 7.3).

PLATELETS

Platelets are seen more frequently in other types of aspirates than in those from the breast. I have no good explanation for this. They appear as small aggregates of light pink irregular fragments, about two to three microns in diameter (Fig. 7.4; Color Plate II).

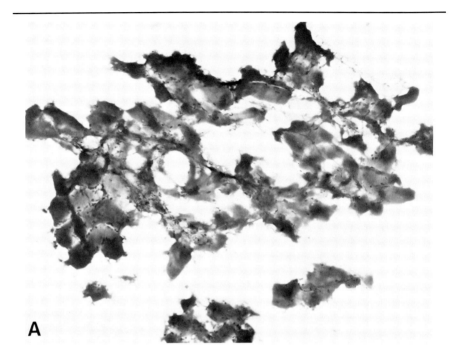

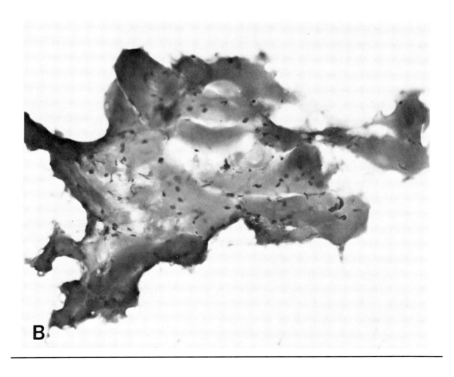

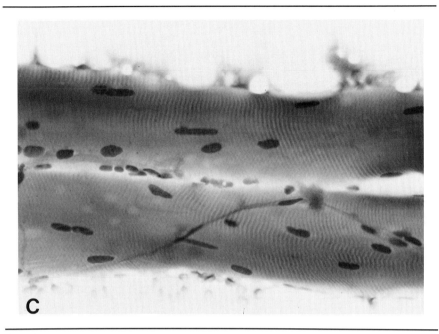

Figure 7.1.
Skeletal muscle. A. (×100). B. (×200). C. (×400).

Figure 7.2.
Fragment of skin. Notice stratum corneum (arrow) *(×100).*

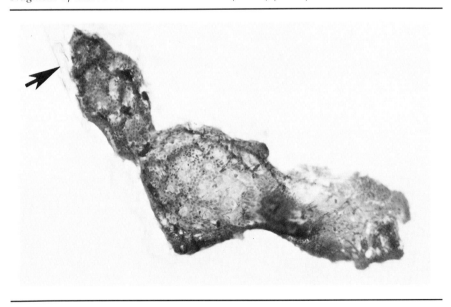

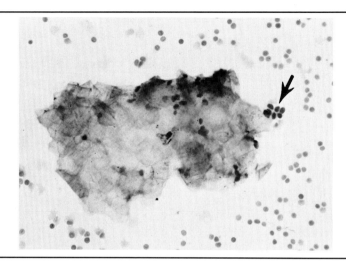

Figure 7.3.
Large cluster of anucleated squamous cells. Note small group of ductal epithelial cells (arrow). Red blood cells are seen in the background (×200).

Figure 7.4.
Ductal epithelial cells and many erythrocytes in the background. Notice two small groups of platelets (arrows) (×400). Inset shows platelets (×750).

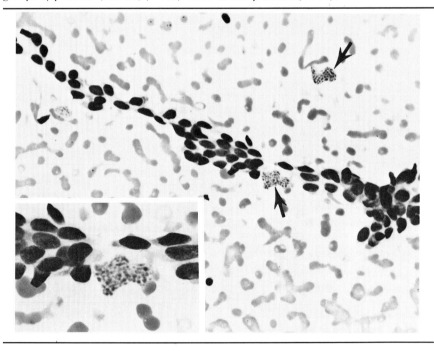

MICROCALCIFICATIONS

Occasionally, in some of the clumps of ductal epithelial cells calcific deposits appear as round, blue-staining, non-birefringent, crystalline material, with a thick border or rim (Fig. 7.5). It is well known that calcifications occur within the breast in both benign (Fig. 7.5) and malignant conditions (Fig. 11.46). It has been reported that 54% of carcinomas and 22% of benign lesions contain calcifications (Snyder and Rosen 1971, p. 1608).

ARTIFACTS

Precipitates of Stain

The most common artifact in breast aspirates is the precipitated dye from the nuclear staining solution (Diff-Quik, solution #2). It has a multilayered appearance and resembles keratin (Figs. 7.6 and 7.7). It can be avoided by keeping the staining dish closed tightly when not in use and also by frequent filtering of the solution. At one time we thought that it represented keratin from the surgeon's hands because, by coincidence, this artifact was much more frequent in those specimens submitted by surgeons.

Figure 7.5.
Microcalcifications. A. Microcalcifications in the center (out of focus) of a cluster of benign ductal epithelial cells (×400). B. Microcalcifications in focus (×400).

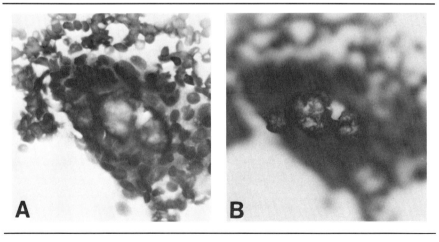

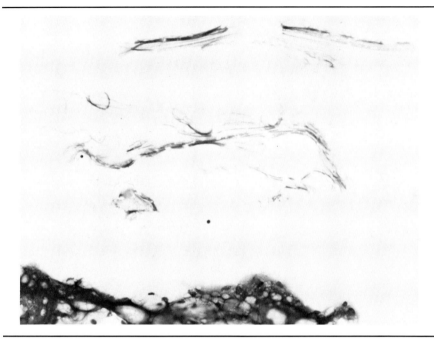

Figure 7.6.
Precipitates of stain and fragment of fibroadipose tissue (×200).

Figure 7.7.
Precipitates of stain (same as in Figure 7.6) resembling layers of keratin (×400).

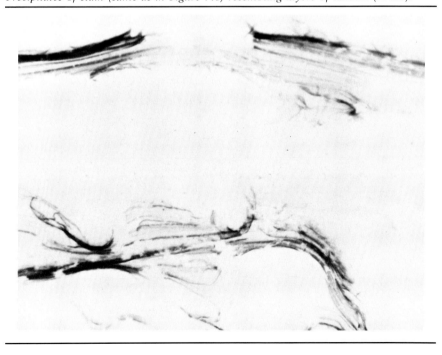

Fernlike Crystals

These crystals are similar to the ferning of the cervical mucus found in vaginal smears. We have observed them only when the specimen has been mixed with saline. Sometimes when the surgeons obtain a dry tap they use a few drops of saline to squirt the scant sample onto the glass slide (Figs. 7.8 and 7.9).

Osmotic Effect on Cells

Osmotic changes are observed in submitted smears. The nuclei appear shaggy, and the cytoplasm either has burst or exploded. This happens when the specimen has been mixed with either saline (Fig. 7.9) or anesthetic fluid.

Cellulose Fibers

Cellulose fibers are seen most often in submitted smears and may obscure cellular detail. The most frequent cause is improper cleaning of glass slides or hemacytometer cover glasses. The source may be gauze, cotton, and paper used to wipe the slides. The fibers stain in shades of blue with the Diff-Quik if they are

Figure 7.8.
Fernlike crystals (×100).

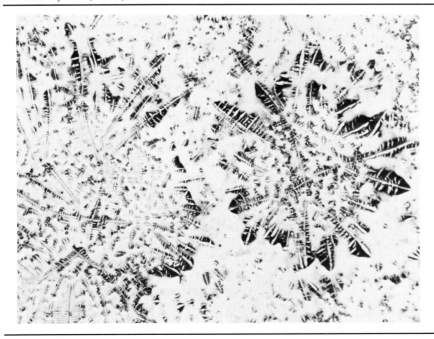

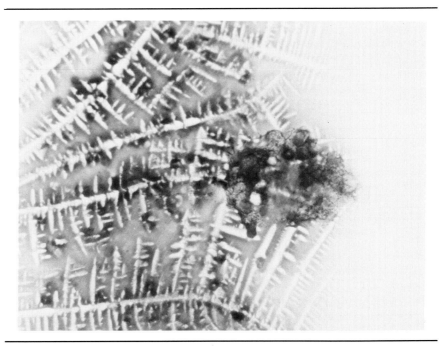

Figure 7.9.
Fernlike crystals and cluster of "exploded" ductal cells (×400).

present on the slide before the smear is made or if they become attached to it while air-drying (Fig. 7.10). They will be seen unstained when deposited on the smears before coverslipping. Although less obtrusive in the last instance, they become more conspicuous under polarized light (Fig. 7.11).

Starch Granules

Starch granules are seen in smears submitted by physicians who wear gloves when they perform an aspiration. They are inconspicuous when in small groups, but occasionally form large clusters (Fig. 7.12). The shape of the granules varies from round to predominantly angular. They stain pale pink or pale blue with a dark blue rim and a yellowish center. Under polarized light the characteristic "maltese crosses" are seen (Fig. 7.13).

Sclereids

Sclereids or stone cells are found in the leaves and stems of many plants. There are four types (Fahn 1974) but we have seen only one variant: the asterosclereids (Fig. 7.14). They have a fenestrated center and small blunt tentacles or protru-

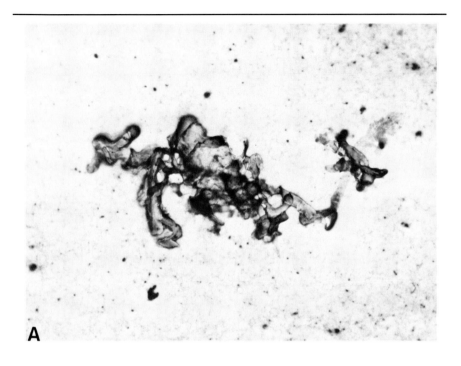

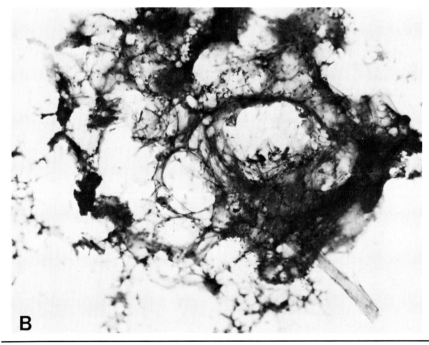

Figure 7.10.
Stained cellulose fibers. A. Large clumps of fibers (×100). B. Fibroadipose tissue and protruding cellulose fiber (×100).

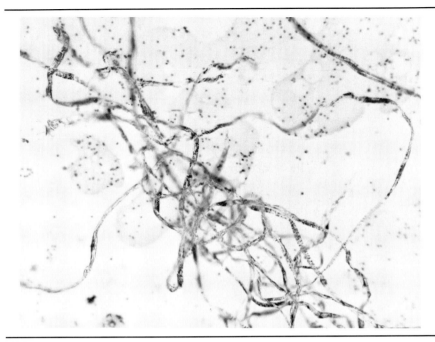

Figure 7.11.
Unstained cellulose fibers from gauze photographed with polarized light (×100).

Figure 7.12.
Starch granules and some erythrocytes in the background (×400).

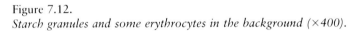

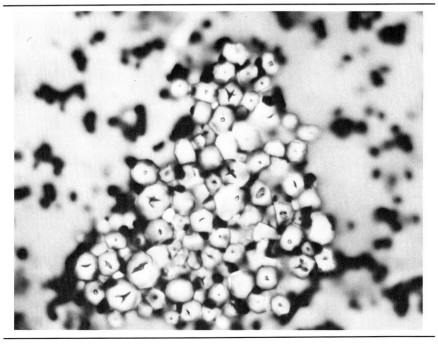

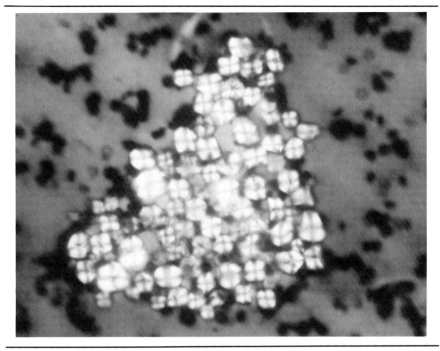

Figure 7.13.
Starch granules (same as in Figure 7.12) photographed with polarized light (×400).

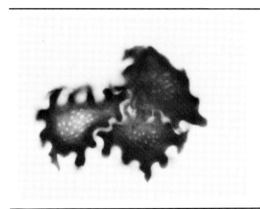

Figure 7.14.
Sclereids or stone cells (×400).

sions; they stain deep blue or bluish green. Sclereids may be observed not only in breast aspirates but in every kind of cytologic smear. I learned of their origin from Dr. B. Naylor in 1981.

Miscellaneous

Other artifacts, such as other plant cells and pollen grains, are seen occasionally.

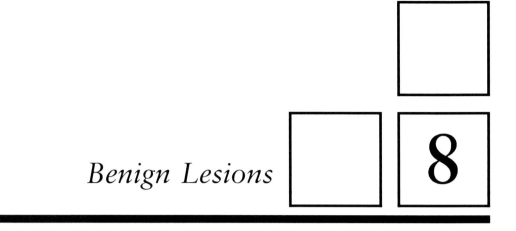

Benign Lesions 8

NON-NEOPLASTIC DISORDERS

Cysts

We share the opinion of those pathologists and clinicians who discourage the processing of fluid from cysts. It is extremely rare to find malignant cells in the fluid aspirated from a cyst. When a cyst is associated with cancer, reaspiration of the residual nodule or lesion will yield the diagnostic cells. As we have mentioned before, draining a breast cyst is not considered a "true aspiration" in our service.

Fibrocystic Disease

The aspirated material is thin and colorless. The smears reveal fragments of fibroadipose tissue, some clusters of benign ductal cells, and clumps of apocrine metaplastic cells. The pathologist also may see histiocytes, stripped nuclei, and oleic acid crystals. To make this diagnosis, apocrine metaplastic cells must be present (Fig. 6.9). In addition, when sheets and clusters of ductal epithelial cells are conspicuous, we diagnose fibrocystic disease with ductal hyperplasia or ductal papillomatosis.

Ductal Hyperplasia (Papillomatosis)

When the smears show many large sheets or monolayers of ductal epithelial cells with folding (Fig. 8.1A), or irregularly shaped clumps with superimposed cells several layers thick forming fingerlike projections and glandular lumina (Fig. 8.1B), we make the diagnosis of ductal hyperplasia or ductal papillomatosis. Some of these groups may contain myoepithelial cells and an occasional nucleus may appear enlarged (Fig. 8.2). This nuclear variation should not cause concern and thus can be ignored. Stripped nuclei are evident in the background.

Squamous Metaplasia

This transformation of glandular epithelium to keratinized epithelium has been reported frequently in the uterine cervix and the tracheobronchial tree, but has received little notice with regard to the breast. Usually it is found in association with fibrocystic disease. The ductal cells appear to undergo squamous change (Fig. 8.3), or some sheets of apocrine cells contain a few cells with abundant dense cytoplasm with angular borders (Fig. 8.4). At low magnification there is a striking difference between the normal ductal epithelial cells and the sheets or groups of squamous metaplastic cells (Fig. 8.3; Color Plate III). Some cells have large nuclei with delicate chromatin and prominent nucleoli. The cytoplasm is very abundant, fairly dense in the paranuclear area, and more delicate toward the edge of the cells. Keratohyaline granules are observed (Fig. 8.5). Some of the nuclei degenerate to ghosts (Fig. 8.6). Some cells may have atypical nuclei and thus be a cause of unnecessary concern (Fig. 8.7).

Sclerosing Adenosis

We believe that sclerosing adenosis is a histologic diagnosis and we do not make this interpretation cytologically.

Ductal Ectasia

The aspirated material from ectatic ducts appears milky, and the smears show many foamy histiocytes (Fig. 8.8). Most are mononuclear histiocytes, but some multinucleated histiocytes are also present. The cytoplasm of the latter contains vacuoles of variable sizes. Also variable are the number and arrangement of nuclei (Fig. 8.9).

Comedomastitis

Clinically comedomastitis can mimic adenocarcinoma and patients may even exhibit peau d'orange. Necrotic debris, hemosiderin-laden macrophages, fibrin

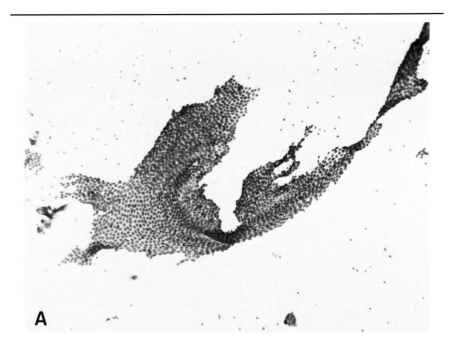

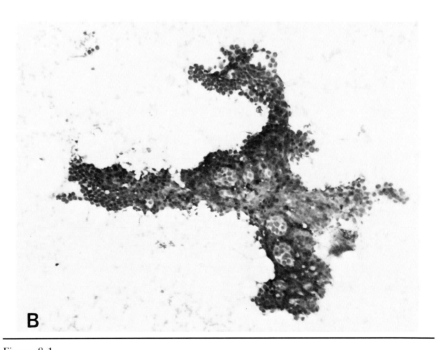

Figure 8.1.
Ductal hyperplasia. A. Large sheet of ductal epithelial cells (×100). B. Irregular, thick clump of ductal cells with fingerlike projections (×100).

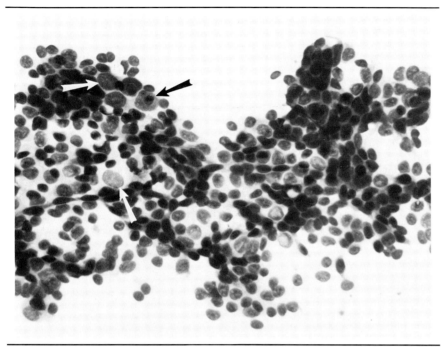

Figure 8.2.
Ductal hyperplasia. Clump of ductal cells, a few with enlarged nuclei (arrows), *and myoepithelial cells (darker and elongated nuclei) (×400).*

Figure 8.3.
Many squamous metaplastic cells (some multinucleated) and small groups of normal ductal cells (×200).

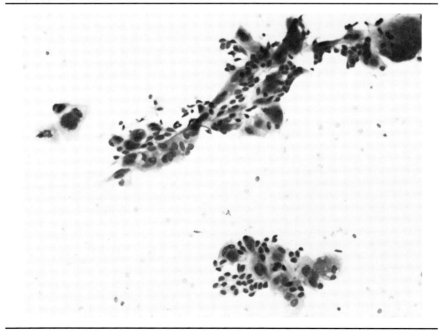

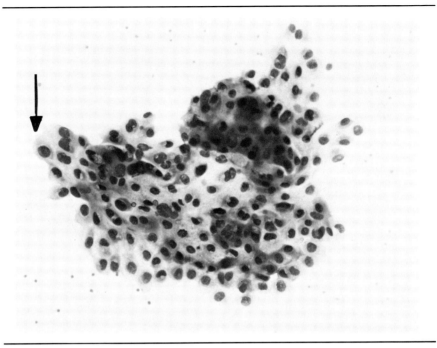

Figure 8.4.
Apocrine metaplastic cells with a few peripheral cells that have undergone some squamous change (arrow) *(×200).*

Figure 8.5.
Small group of squamous metaplastic cells with abundant cytoplasm with keratohyalin granules, ovoid nuclei, and conspicuous nucleoli (×400).

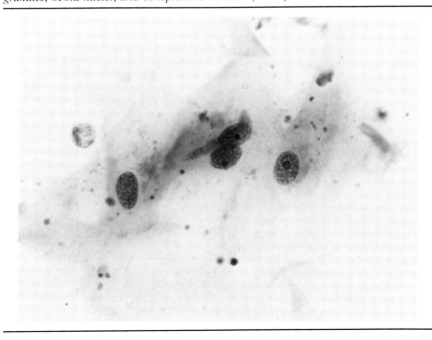

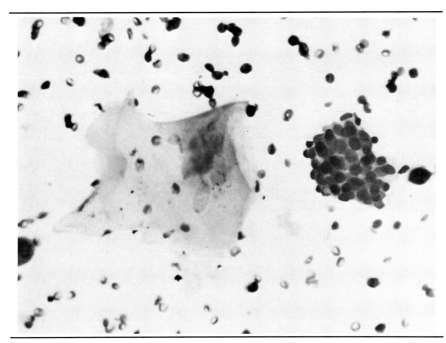

Figure 8.6.
Squamous metaplastic cells with ghost nuclei and a cluster of benign ductal epithelial cells (×400).

Figure 8.7.
Squamous metaplastic cells with nuclear atypia. A. (×400). B. (×400).

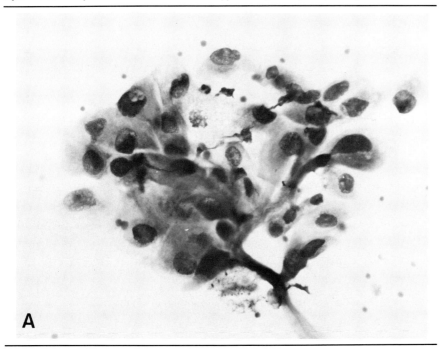

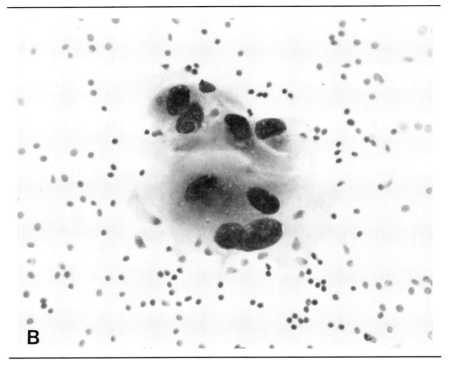

Figure 8.7.
(continued)

Figure 8.8.
Ductal ectasia. Many foamy histiocytes and a cluster of ductal epithelial cells (×400).

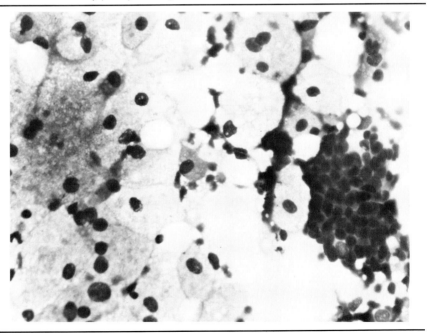

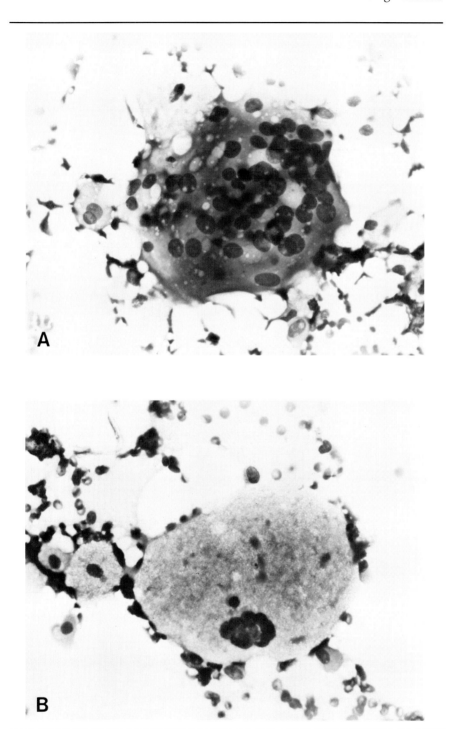

Figure 8.9.
Ductal ectasia: multinucleated histiocytes. A. Many nuclei irregularly distributed in the dense cytoplasm (×400). B. Several mononuclear histiocytes surround a large multinucleated histiocyte in which the nuclei are tightly clumped (×400).

strands, and some clumps of epithelial cells are seen. Some of these cells may show slight nuclear irregularity (Fig. 8.10); however, we have noticed many dark blue granules in their cytoplasm (Figs. 8.10B and 8.11). Comedocarcinoma has to be considered in the differential diagnosis; we will discuss these aspects in more detail in Chapter 15 on pitfalls. We have noticed also the presence of abundant acellular proteinaceous material, staining pale blue and adopting variable shapes (some round, but predominantly with an ovoid configuration) (Fig. 8.12).

Fibrous Mastopathy

Fibrous mastopathy can be considered that part of the spectrum of fibrocystic disease composed exclusively of the stromal or fibrous component. The lesion is moderately firm and offers a rubbery resistance to the needle. Smears are scant with occasional fragments of adipose and fibrous tissue in addition to a few ductal cells (Figs. 8.13 and 8.14).

Fatty Replacement

Abundant mature fibroadipose tissue, similar to that described previously, is observed (Fig. 6.1).

Figure 8.10.
Comedomastitis. A. Large irregular clump of ductal epithelial cells with some enlarged nuclei (arrow) *(×100). B. Enlargement of A (×400).*

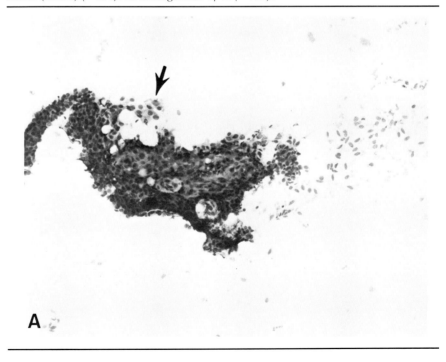

A

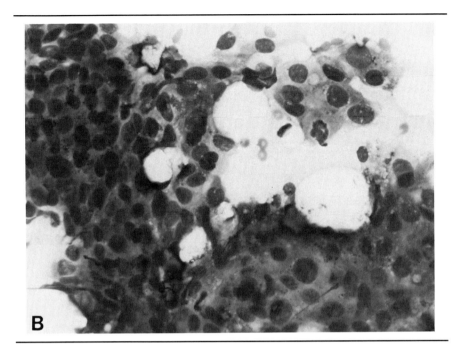

Figure 8.11.
Comedomastitis. Clump of ductal epithelial cells with variation in nuclear size and a few fine cytoplasmic granules (arrows) *(×400).*

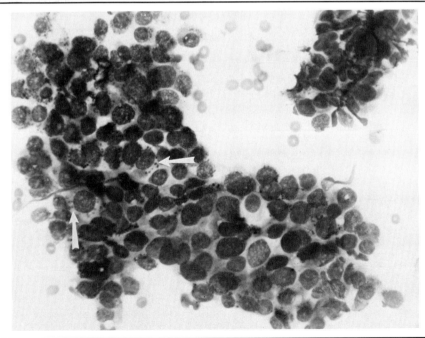

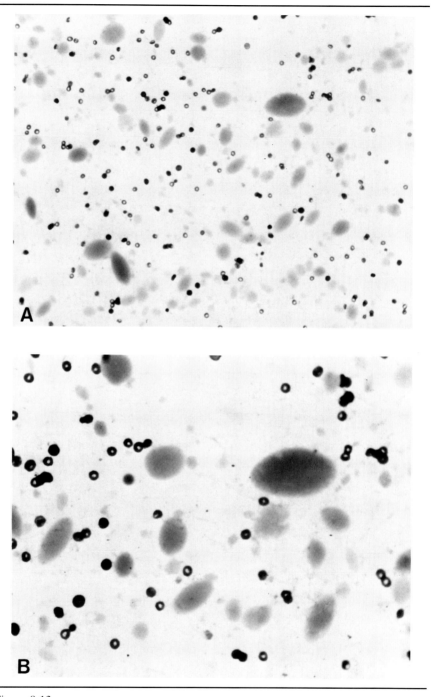

Figure 8.12.
Comedomastitis: ovoid proteinaceous material. A. (×200). B. (×400).

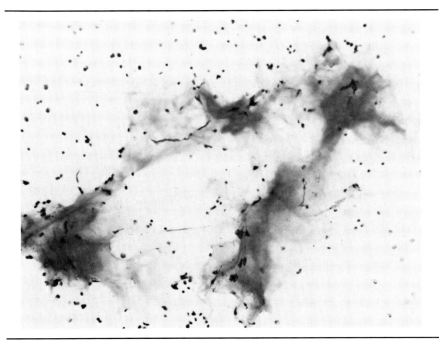

Figure 8.13.
Fibrous mastopathy. Irregular fragments of sparsely cellular fibrous tissue (×200).

Figure 8.14.
Fibrous mastopathy. Clumps of ductal epithelial cells and fibroblasts with stringy cytoplasm (×400).

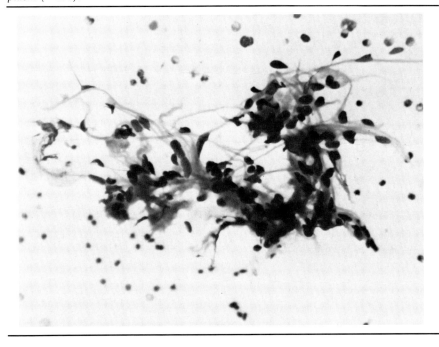

LESIONS SECONDARY TO TRAUMA

Fat Necrosis

To the naked eye, these smears tend to be fairly thick and granular. Under low power, vacuoles of variable sizes are seen. Higher magnification reveals that these "vacuoles" (in fact, adipocytes) may or may not have nuclei. Variable numbers of acute inflammatory cells are present. Some histiocytes (a few multi-nucleated), lymphocytes, and plasma cells also are seen (Fig. 8.15). Newly formed capillaries in addition to clumps of ductal cells are seen in some cases. Some degree of nuclear atypia is to be expected. Further detail will be given in Chapter 15.

Organizing Hematoma

Organizing hematoma may present as a discrete mass. The patient may or may not be aware of previous trauma. Cytologically, large numbers of cholesterol crystals are observed, but these easily may be overlooked or interpreted as an artifact at low magnification (Fig. 8.16). It is only at higher magnification that the stacks of rhomboid crystals are identified; often each crystal has a corner missing (Fig. 8.17). Variable numbers of hemosiderin-laden macrophages and multinucleated giant cells are observed. In other instances lysed blood and some plump fibroblasts predominate. The latter can adopt bizarre shapes and have large nuclei and prominent nucleoli (Fig. 15.1; Color Plate IV). They are a source of false positive diagnosis, as we will discuss in Chapter 15.

HORMONAL CHANGES

Lactation

At low power the smears appear bubbly, have proteinaceous fluid in the background, and usually scant cellularity (Fig. 8.18). Some single epithelial cells and enlarged and irregular naked nuclei with easily detected nucleoli are present. Other cells are in sheets, in thick clumps, or are arranged in syncytial clusters with ill-defined cell borders (Fig. 8.19). Most of them show marked cytoplasmic fragility and crush artifact. The better preserved cytoplasm contains bluish granules and many vacuoles, which seem to be more numerous at the periphery of the clumps. The nuclei have prominent nucleoli (one or two per nucleus) and some vacuoles. Variable numbers of foamy histiocytes are present and connective tissue fragments appear loose and more cellular (see Color Plates V and VI).

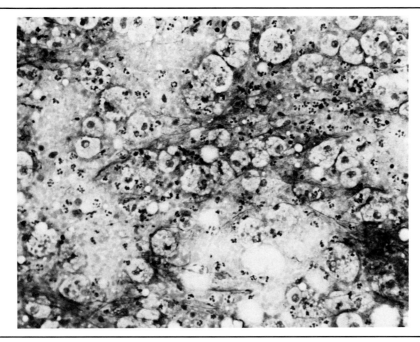

Figure 8.15.
Fat necrosis. Many polymorphonuclear leukocytes and foamy histiocytes. Foci like this are also seen in cases of acute and chronic mastitis (×200).

Figure 8.16.
Organizing hematoma. The numerous clear, angular spaces represent cholesterol crystals that can be easily overlooked at this low magnification (×100).

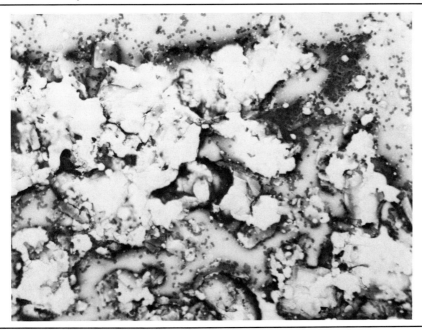

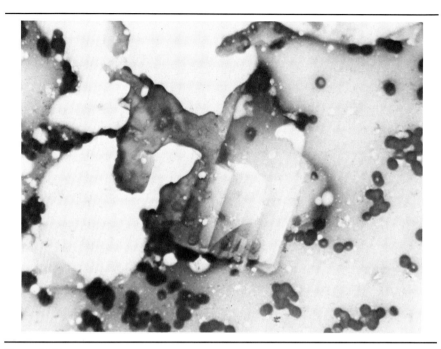

Figure 8.17.
Organizing hematoma. Stacked cholesterol crystals lie in the center of the field (×400).

Figure 8.18.
Lactation. Notice proteinaceous bubbly background (×200).

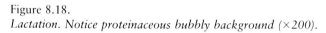

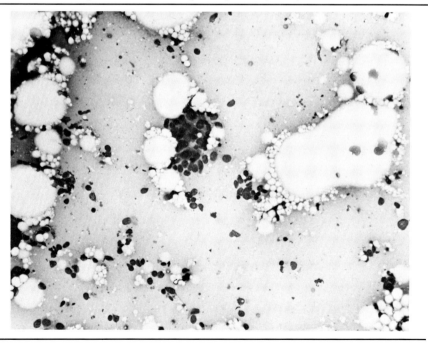

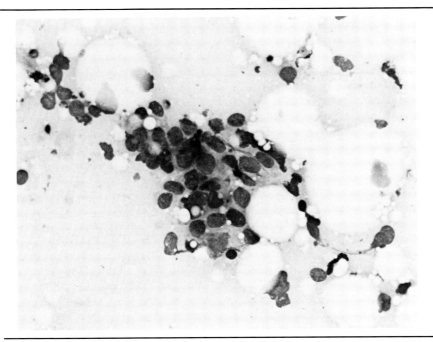

Figure 8.19.
Lactation. Groups of ductal cells with poorly demarcated cell borders and cytoplasmic and nuclear vacuoles (×400).

BACTERIAL AND VIRAL DISEASES

Acute Mastitis or Abscess

The smears tend to be fairly thick and when studied under the microscope show large numbers of polymorphonuclear leukocytes and fibrin strands (Fig. 8.20), some cellular debris, foamy histiocytes, and occasional ductal cells. In some instances the ductal epithelial cells appear markedly atypical and lead to diagnostic difficulties (see Chapter 15 and Color Plate VII).

Subareolar Abscess

Under low magnification the smears are reminiscent of an acute mastitis or abscess. However, in a background of inflammatory cells, well-defined clear or pale blue spaces that correspond to anucleated squames are observed (Fig. 8.21; Color Plates VIII and IX). In some areas of the smear there are large clusters of squamous epithelial cells; in these the cell borders are more evident and occasional nuclei may be observed (Fig. 8.22). Foamy histiocytes, lymphocytes, plasma cells, and some capillaries are also present (Fig. 8.21; Color Plate VIII). Multinucleated giant cells are seen in the vicinity of the capillaries. For additional information refer to the work of Galblum and Oertel (1983).

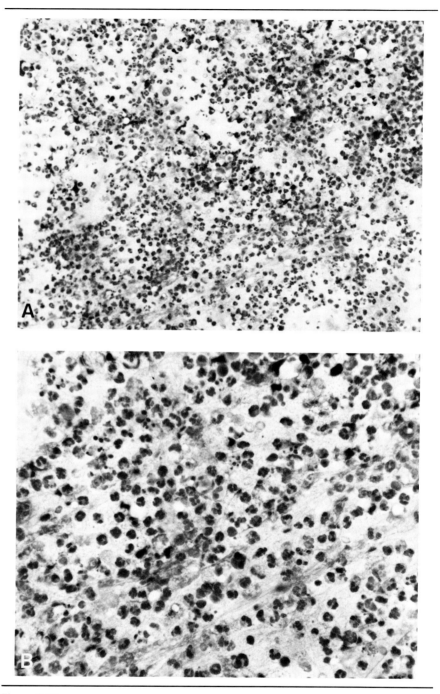

Figure 8.20.
Acute mastitis. A. *Extremely cellular smear (×200).* B. *Fibrin strands and many polymor-phonuclear leukocytes are readily identified (×400).*

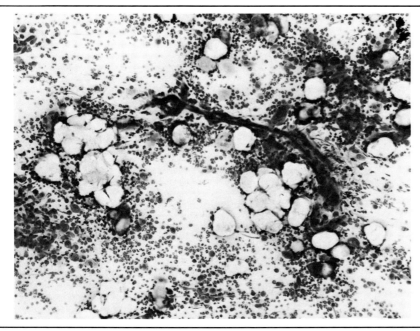

Figure 8.21.
Subareolar abscess. Very cellular smears with inflammatory cells and many anucleated squames (some in large clusters). Notice the branching capillary (×100).

Figure 8.22.
Subareolar abscess. The clear angulated spaces correspond to anucleated squamous cells surrounded by polymorphonuclear leukocytes. To the left a thick clump of keratinized cells with dense cytoplasm and a few with hyperchromatic nuclei (×200).

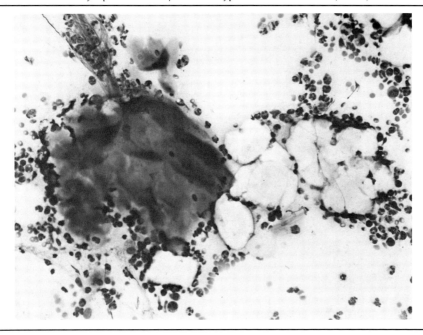

Granulomatous Mastitis

Most frequently this condition will be a reaction to suture material (foreign-body granulomata) following an excisional biopsy. Physical examination will reveal a nodule or lump underlying a surgical scar. Fragments of fibrous tissue and some epithelioid and multinucleated giant cells are seen. Sometimes birefringent material can be observed in the cytoplasm of the latter (Color Plate X). We also have had one case of tuberculous granulomatous mastitis, clinically suspected to be a carcinoma. Vassilakos (1973) reported a similar experience. Under low magnification the smears are very cellular (Fig. 8.23), and the possibility of a neoplasm must be considered; some of the cells are arranged in clusters and others are seen lying singly. Under higher magnification the cell clusters are thick and fairly cohesive, and there is marked cellular superimposition. The predominant cells have elongated, cigar-shaped nuclei with poorly defined cytoplasmic borders (Fig. 8.24). Other cells have round nuclei, and occasionally a multinucleated giant cell can be observed. In other areas of the smear the groups consist of occasional epithelioid cells and cells believed to be reactive ductal cells with enlarged, atypical nuclei. The cellular atypia can be remarkable when compared with adjacent, apparently normal ductal cells (Fig. 8.25).

Additional cases of tuberculous mastitis, diagnosed by fine needle aspiration, have been reported recently from India (Nayar and Saxena 1984; Jayaram 1985).

Herpesvirus Infection

Although not an aspiration, we feel prompted to discuss this case because clinically it was interpreted as Paget's disease of the breast. A 38-year-old white woman presented with an eroded lesion of the nipple, with oozing and crusting. In addition she had a palpable, ipsilateral axillary lymph node. Touch preparations from the nipple showed large numbers of inflammatory cells (polymorphonuclear leukocytes and some lymphoid cells) and numerous markedly atypical epithelial cells, singly and in clusters (Fig. 8.26). At higher magnification, some of the single cells were round, had a high nuclear/cytoplasmic ratio and a small rim of cytoplasm (Fig. 8.27). Others were multinucleated and irregular in shape (Fig. 8.28). To inexperienced eyes the lesion was interpreted as a poorly differentiated carcinoma. Detailed examination of the cells revealed large nuclei resembling "stacks of poker chips," that showed margination of the nuclear chromatin (Figs. 8.28 and 8.29). No intranuclear inclusions were seen. The fine needle aspiration from the palpable axillary node did not reveal any evidence of metastasis, but rather a reactive lymphadenopathy secondary to the viral infection. The lesion resolved in two weeks.

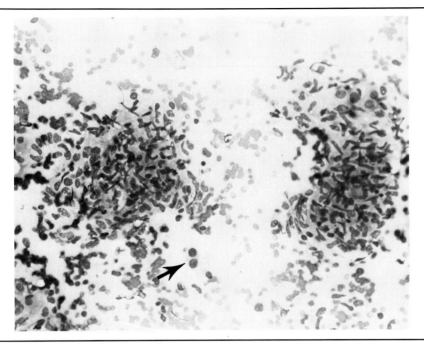

Figure 8.23.
Tuberculous granulomatous mastitis. Large clumps of cells and some isolated cells (arrow) *with enlarged nuclei (compare to size of erythrocytes in the background) (×200).*

Figure 8.24.
Tuberculous granulomatous mastitis. Granuloma with epithelioid cells (elongated nuclei) and multinucleated cell (arrow) *(×400).*

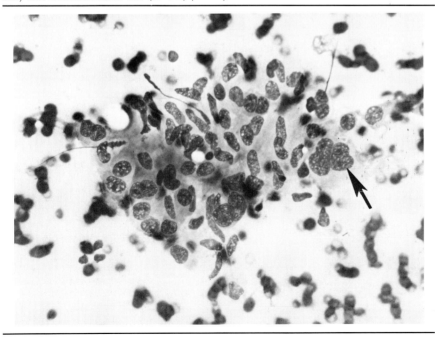

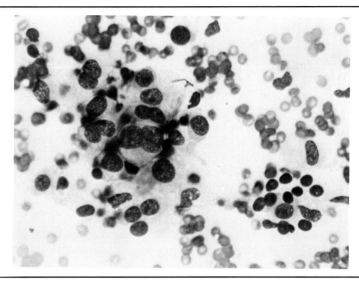

Figure 8.25.
Tuberculous granulomatous mastitis. Ductal cells with enlarged nuclei and a small group of loosely cohesive normal ductal cells (×400).

Figure 8.26.
Herpesvirus infection. Very cellular smears with large clumps of cells and some isolated cells (×100).

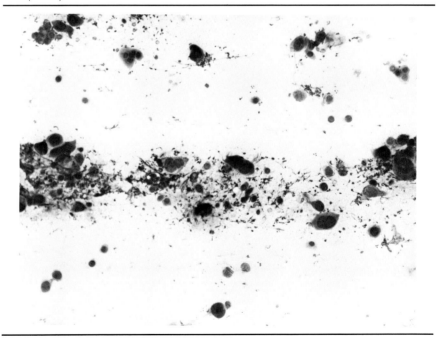

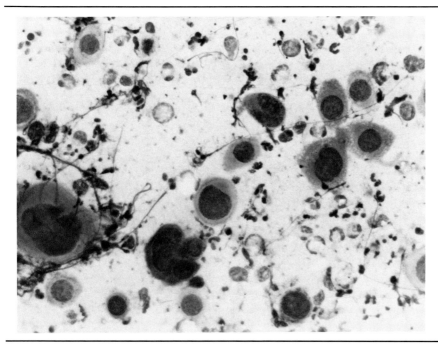

Figure 8.27.
Herpesvirus infection. Round cells (one very large and bizarre) with high nuclear/ cytoplasmic ratio and numerous inflammatory cells (×400).

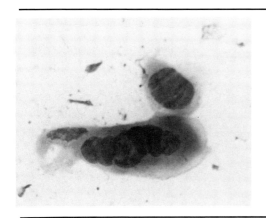

Figure 8.28.
Two large multinucleated epithelial cells characteristic of herpesvirus infection. Note "stacked nuclei" (×400).

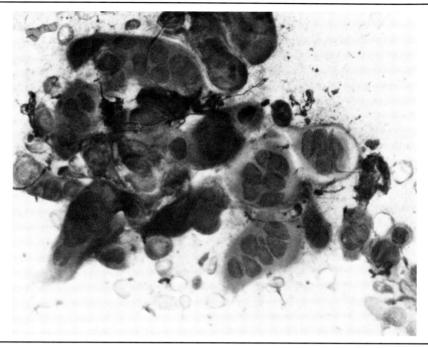

Figure 8.29.
Clump of multinucleated epithelial cells typical of herpesvirus infection (×400).

BENIGN NEOPLASMS

Fibroadenoma

Fibroadenoma presents as a discrete nodule that is rubbery on aspiration. Smears from these lesions are quite cellular and are the leading cause of false positive diagnosis. I believe "pattern recognition" is extremely important (Color Plates XI and XII). The presence of abundant bright pink fibrous connective tissue fragments is the hallmark of the lesion (Fig. 8.30; Color Plate XIII). However, in submitted smears the most frequent pattern is the presence of many cohesive ductal epithelial cells arranged in extremely large sheets and clusters of variable shapes (Fig. 8.31). In the background there are many loose cells. At higher magnification a few nuclei and occasional blood vessels are found in the fibrous connective tissue. The sheets of epithelial cells have a honeycomb appearance with somewhat enlarged but regular nuclei and scant to moderate cytoplasm. Folding of these monolayers of ductal cells is common (Figs. 8.32 and 8.33). Some clumps have a three-dimensional appearance, with well-demarcated rounded borders known as blunt branching (Figs. 8.34 and 8.35). Occupying the background, between the sheets of epithelial cells, are some single cells and many ovoid naked nuclei (Figs. 8.34 and 8.36A)—the bipolar

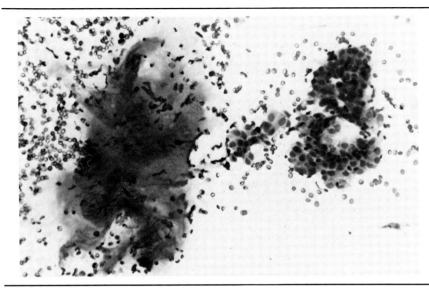

Figure 8.30.
Fibroadenoma. Fragment of fibrous connective tissue and clump of ductal cells (×200).

Figure 8.31.
Fibroadenoma. Extremely large, irregular, tightly cohesive clusters of ductal cells (×40).

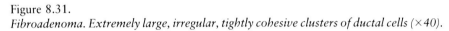

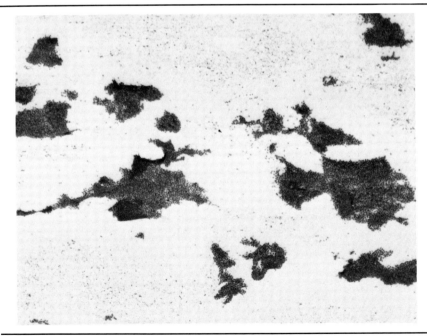

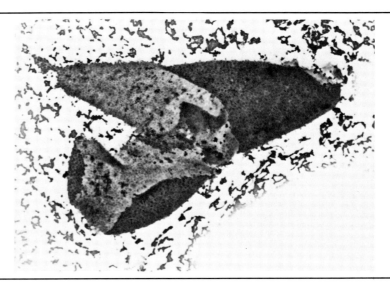

Figure 8.32.
Fibroadenoma. Folded sheet of ductal cells (×100).

Figure 8.33.
Fibroadenoma. Folded sheet of ductal cells (×200).

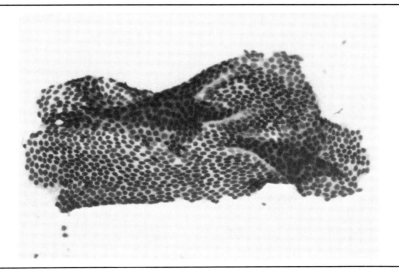

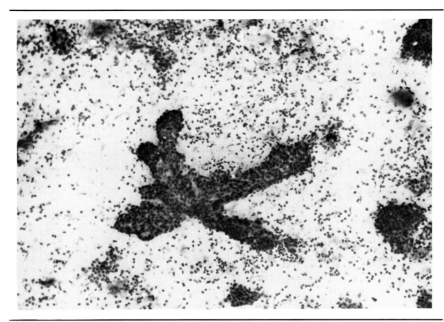

Figure 8.34.
Fibroadenoma. Blunt branching of epithelial cells and bipolar stripped nuclei in the background (×100).

Figure 8.35.
Fibroadenoma. Blunt branching (×200).

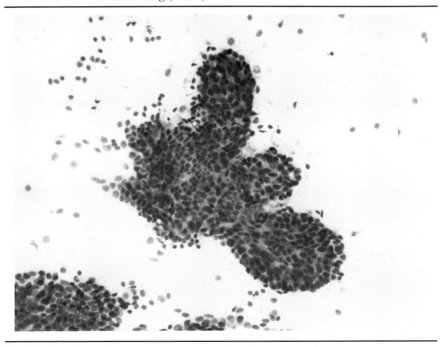

stripped nuclei discussed in the Swedish literature. Some pathologists believe that they represent myoepithelial cells while others think that they represent fibroblasts. Occasional intranuclear inclusions are seen (Figs. 8.36B–D). Some of the single cells seen in the background have scant, elongated, pale blue cytoplasm, ovoid nuclei, and *occasional* nucleoli visible. A few groups of apocrine metaplastic cells may be observed in some cases, as may foamy histiocytes (mononucleated and multinucleated). Once the pattern of fibroadenoma is recognized under low magnification, one should not spend much time analyzing the variation in the size of the nuclei; it leads to unnecessary worry. It might be argued that one might miss a carcinoma associated with the fibroadenoma. We should remember that this association is rare. In addition, when a carcinoma is present, it is usually of the lobular type. In any event, the fibroadenoma will have to be excised.

It has been claimed that it is difficult to differentiate between a fibroadenoma and fibrocystic disease and/or mammary dysplasia (Linsk et al 1972). This is a frequent occurrence when dealing with submitted smears. If the pathologist

Figure 8.36.
Fibroadenoma. A. Bipolar stripped nuclei (×1000). B and C. Intranuclear inclusions, representing evaginations of the cytoplasm (probably of epithelial cell) into the nucleus (×1000). D. Pseudo intranuclear inclusion. This is most likely an artifact since the nucleus is small and the inclusion is too homogeneous and clear (×1000).

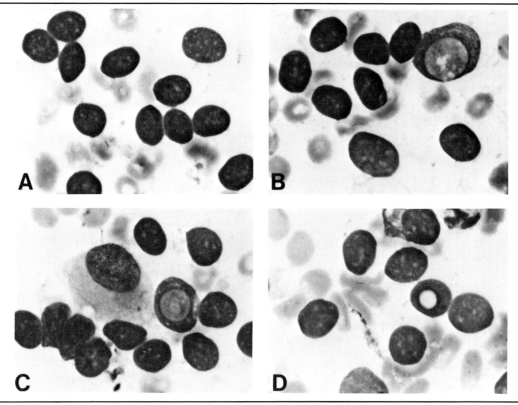

performs the aspiration, it will happen less often. Table 8.1 lists the criteria for differential diagnosis. As both lesions are benign, this is purely of academic interest.

Lipoma

Cytologically the findings in lipoma are identical to those described in fatty replacement (Fig. 6.1). If the pathologist is performing the aspiration, clinical differentiation between the two entities is likely. A lipoma is palpated as a discrete, soft mass. In the case of fatty replacement, there is no discrete lesion.

Papilloma

When a papilloma is present, the patient will complain most frequently of a hemorrhagic discharge from the nipple. Examination of the smears may reveal hemosiderin-laden macrophages and a few clusters of ductal cells with a moderate amount of cytoplasm. If a lesion is palpated, the aspirate usually yields some hemorrhagic or lightly blood-tinged fluid. Depending on the amount and consistency of the fluid aspirated, direct smears or smears from the sediment of the fluid can be prepared. They demonstrate a proteinaceous background with some amorphous debris, some erythrocytes, some hemosiderin-laden macro-

Table 8.1
Diagnostic criteria to differentiate between fibroadenoma and fibrocystic disease

Criteria	Fibroadenoma	Fibrocystic Disease
Tumor cellularity.	Present.	Very seldom seen.
Sheets of cells.	Numerous.	Less frequent.
Clumps of cells.	Many with blunt branching; some irregular tissue fragments.	Some with blunt branching; many small irregular tissue fragments.
Apocrine cells.	Rare.	Very numerous.
Naked nuclei.	Innumerable.	Some.
Fibrous tissue.	Very abundant, large fragments staining bright pink.	Scant to moderate, small fragments.
Foamy histiocytes.	Occasional.	Many.
Adipose tissue.	Absent.	Present.
Findings on palpation and during aspiration.	Discrete mass; does not "disappear" on aspiration; rubbery.	Ill-defined "lumps"; discrete "cysts" that collapse on aspiration. Softer; variable amounts of fluid.

phages (mononucleated and multinucleated), and a few inflammatory cells. There are also small clusters of ductal cells with slightly enlarged nuclei and with some variation in nuclear size and shape; a moderate amount of cytoplasm is present that becomes extremely attenuated and clear in some of the cells located at the edges of the clump (Figs. 8.37–8.39). Sometimes a few small clusters of ductal epithelial cells are attached to loose, granular connective tissue that appears degenerated (Fig. 8.40). In general, the smears are hypocellular and the clusters of cells are relatively small when compared to those of fibroadenoma.

Granular Cell Tumor

Clinically it resembles mammary carcinoma. The lesion is firm, ill-defined, and occasionally causes skin retraction. There is resistance to the needle though it is not gritty on aspiration. The smears can be extremely cellular. The well-preserved cells have enlarged nuclei with prominent nucleoli and cytoplasm in which dense regions alternate with vacuolated areas (Figs. 8.41–8.43). The granularity of the cytoplasm is more evident in alcohol-fixed, Papanicolaou-stained material.

The cellular fragility is remarkable. Extra care has to be applied when making the smears; if not, the cytoplasm of most cells will be destroyed, and all you will observe are naked nuclei in a dirty granular background (Color Plates XIV and

Figure 8.37.
Papilloma. Two clusters of ductal cells in a hemorrhagic background. Note hemosiderin-laden macrophages (×200).

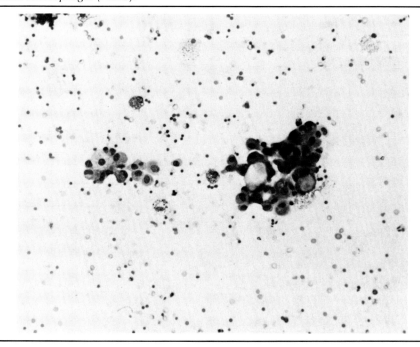

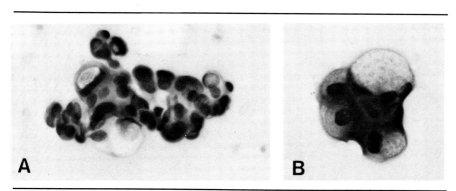

Figure 8.38.
Papilloma. A *and* B. *Two small epithelial clusters showing cytoplasmic clearing (×400).*

Figure 8.39.
Papilloma. A group of epithelial cells with cytoplasmic clearing (×1000).

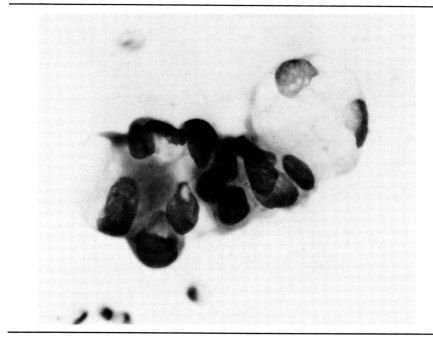

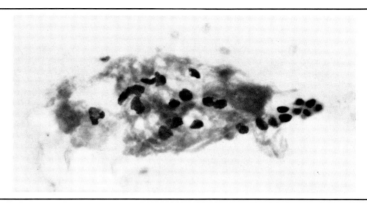

Figure 8.40.
Papilloma. Small groups of ductal cells embedded in loose connective tissue (×400).

Figure 8.41.
Granular cell myoblastoma. Cellular smears showing clusters of cells and some isolated cells. The cytoplasm varies in density (×200).

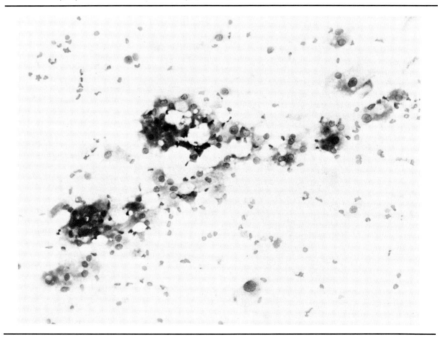

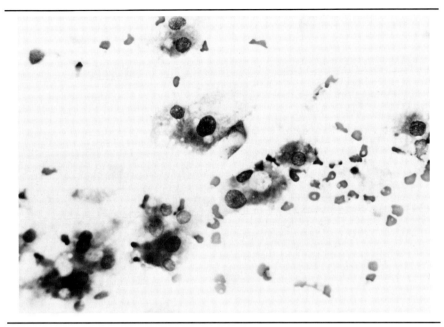

Figure 8.42.
Granular cell myoblastoma. Loosely cohesive cells with moderately well preserved cytoplasm of variable density. Two nuclei display conspicuous nucleoli (×400).

Figure 8.43.
Granular cell myoblastoma. The cytoplasm of these cells varies from pale and attenuated to dense to coarsely granular (×400).

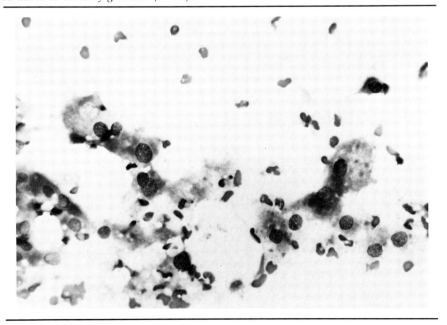

XV). Thus, when the pathologist suspects this entity after reviewing the first prepared slides, an especially careful technique can be applied to obtain intact cells.

Löwhagen and Rubio (1977, p. 315) reported "cells having poorly stained nucleus and heavily granular cytoplasm" on May-Grünwald Giemsa-stained smears. This has not been our experience.

Nodular Fasciitis

The lesion is firm and ill defined, and the smears are moderately cellular. There are some cells with plump, ovoid to round nuclei, some prominent nucleoli, and variable amounts of pale blue cytoplasm embedded in irregular fragments of fibrocollagenous tissue (Fig. 8.44). The cells have variable shapes; some are polygonal while others are spindled. There are many single cells with large nuclei, prominent nucleoli, and abundant cytoplasm (Fig. 8.45). This is a rare entity in this location (Fritsches and Muller 1983).

Figure 8.44.
Nodular fasciitis. Cellular smears: some of the cells are loose while others are embedded in dense fibrous tissue (×200).

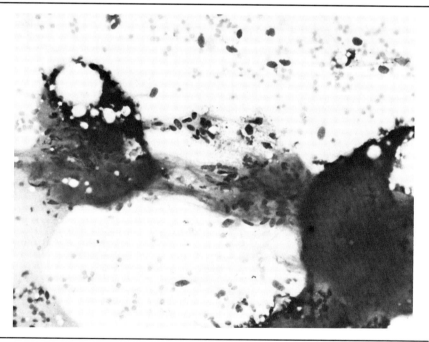

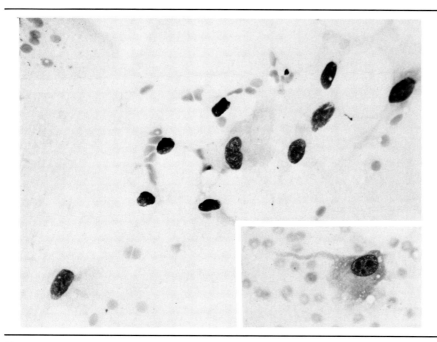

Figure 8.45.
Nodular fasciitis. Some of the loose cells have very delicate and attenuated cytoplasm (×400). Inset shows an atypical cell (×400).

MISCELLANEOUS

Accessory Mammary Tissue in Axilla

Sometimes the patient has been aware, for several years, of an axillary mass that waxes and wanes, particularly in relation to her menses. Other patients notice an axillary lump during the first few months of pregnancy. In the first instance, fine needle aspiration will reveal benign ductal cells with very scanty cytoplasm. In the second instance, the breast tissue will show the characteristic changes of lactation that we have described already in detail. Metastatic breast carcinoma might be considered in the differential diagnosis. Clinically, the patients are younger than the usual patient with breast carcinoma, and no primary lesion is palpated. On aspiration, the lesion is soft and there is no cellular atypia in the smears.

Intramammary Lymph Node

These are discrete, small, firm, usually movable lesions on palpation, more commonly present in the upper outer quadrant, although we also have noted them in the lower outer quadrant. On aspiration they are soft. The smears show

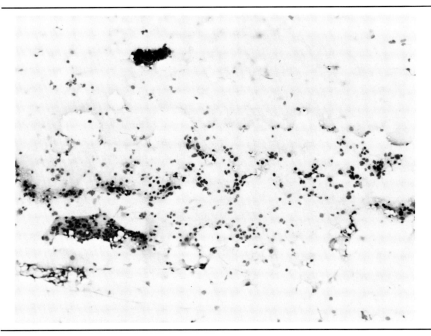

Figure 8.46.
Intramammary lymph node. Moderately cellular smears with a proteinaceous background and numerous small loose cells. A tight cluster of ductal cells is observed in the upper left (×100).

Figure 8.47.
Intramammary lymph node. Small and large lymphocytes (×200).

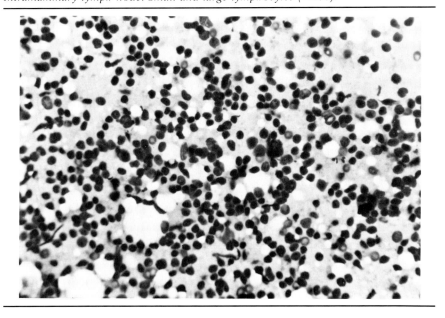

abundant lymphoid tissue consisting of mature lymphocytes and some reticular cells in a proteinaceous background (Figs. 8.46 and 8.47). When the lesion is small, the needle may go through it and also sample normal parenchyma. The smears show an occasional cluster of benign ductal cells (Fig. 8.46).

Gynecomastia

This is one of the few instances in which the procedure can be extremely painful.

The smears are moderately cellular. Many fragments of fibroadipose tissue and numerous small to fairly large cellular clusters are seen (Fig. 8.48) that may

Figure 8.48.
Gynecomastia. Very large, irregular, tightly cohesive fragment of ductal epithelium. Notice the small fragment of fibrocollagenous tissue at the upper right (arrow) (×100).

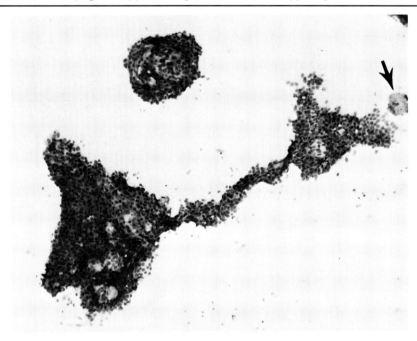

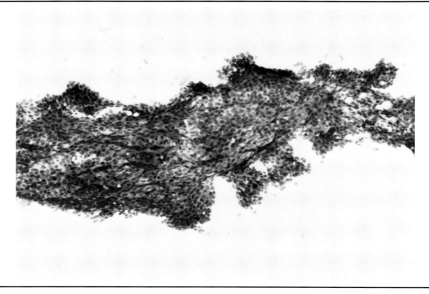

Figure 8.49.
Gynecomastia. Ductal epithelial cells and "streams" of myoepithelial cells (×100).

Figure 8.50.
Gynecomastia. Thick fragment of tissue with regular, round to ovoid ductal epithelial cell nuclei. The myoepithelial cells have darker and more elongated nuclei (×400).

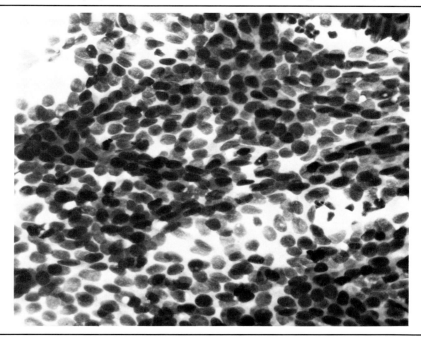

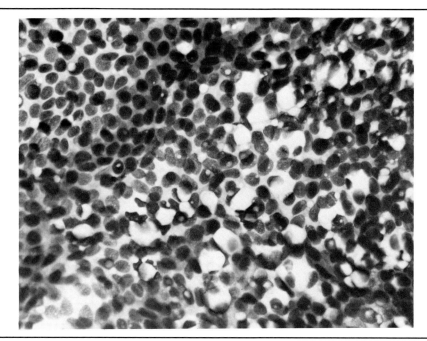

Figure 8.51.
Gynecomastia. In this case the sheet of ductal cells shows marked cytoplasmic vacuolation. Some of the nuclei also have small vacuoles (×400).

show some variation in nuclear size. However, myoepithelial cells are observed (Figs. 8.49 and 8.50). Frequently the sheets of epithelial cells show nuclear and cytoplasmic vacuolation that can be marked (Fig. 8.51). Occasional atypical single cells are present. Stripped bipolar nuclei may be seen in the background. Sometimes apocrine metaplastic cells are observed.

Atypical Ductal Hyperplasia

9

The two principal possibilities with which the pathologist is concerned when examining a smear are whether the changes are benign or malignant. If a good sample has been obtained, the answer will be obvious in most cases. In some cases, however, a conclusion can be reached, but only with difficulty. There always will be a few cases in which doubts will remain regardless of the number of needles inserted and smears prepared. For these cases we reserve the label *atypical hyperplasia.*

DUCTAL HYPERPLASIA OR ATYPICAL DUCTAL HYPERPLASIA?

In ductal hyperplasia (or papillomatosis) the sheets or monolayers of ductal cells are larger than normal and folded (Figs. 8.1 and 8.2). Some groups or clumps exhibit superimposition of cells and a tendency to form fingerlike projections and glandular lumina (Figs. 9.1 and 9.2). Other cells may have enlarged nuclei (Figs. 9.3 and 9.4) and conspicuous nucleoli. Apocrine metaplastic cells, when present, provide some reassurance that the lesion is probably benign. If only an occasional cluster of ductal cells shows some variation in nuclear size, this should raise no concern and can be ignored.

When we make a diagnosis of *atypical* ductal hyperplasia we look for (1) increased overall cellularity (Fig. 9.5) with clumps and loose cells; (2) cells within the clumps and sheets that appear to have lost some of their cohesiveness (Figs. 9.5 and 9.6); (3) moderate nuclear enlargement and variation in nuclear size, both in the clumps (Figs. 9.7–9.10), and in the single cells (Fig. 9.11).

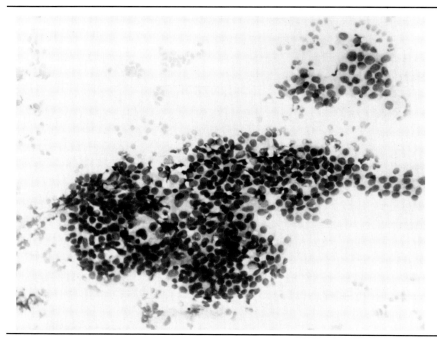

Figure 9.1.
Ductal hyperplasia or papillomatosis. Large irregular clump of cohesive ductal cells (×200).

Figure 9.2.
Ductal hyperplasia. Sheet of ductal cells with myoepithelial cells (darker and elongated nuclei) and with a tendency to form glandular lumina (×400).

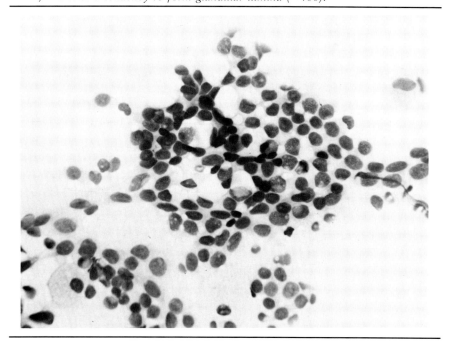

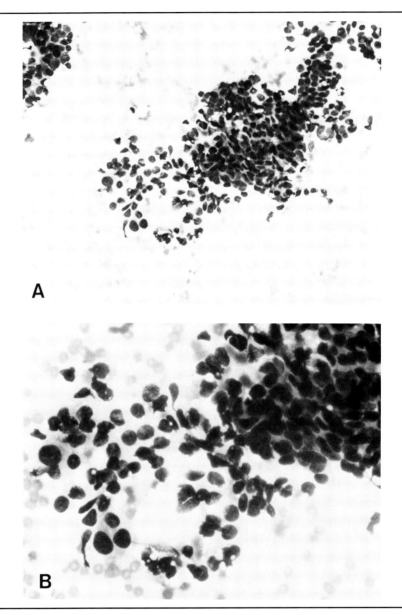

Figure 9.3.
Ductal hyperplasia. Irregular cluster of ductal cells some of which are loosely cohesive and show variation in nuclear size. A (×200). B (×400).

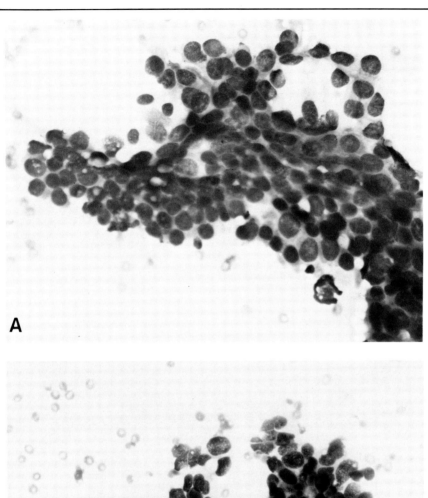

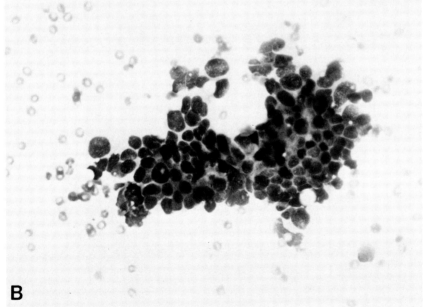

Figure 9.4.
Ductal hyperplasia. Clusters of epithelial cells showing variation in nuclear size (×400).
Note: *If only one or two of these clusters are present per smear we make the diagnosis of ductal hyperplasia. However, when numerous such clusters are present we diagnose atypical ductal hyperplasia.*

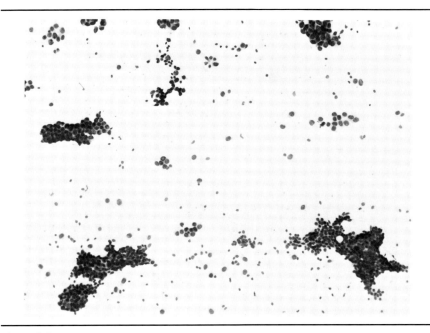

Figure 9.5.
Atypical ductal hyperplasia. Very cellular smears with clumps of epithelial cells and some loose cells (×100). Compare with tumor cellularity seen in Figure 10.1 at same magnification and with Figure 10.3 for size of cellular clusters (also at ×100).

Figure 9.6.
Atypical ductal hyperplasia. Loosely cohesive epithelial cells showing variation in nuclear size. Some bipolar nuclei seen (×200).

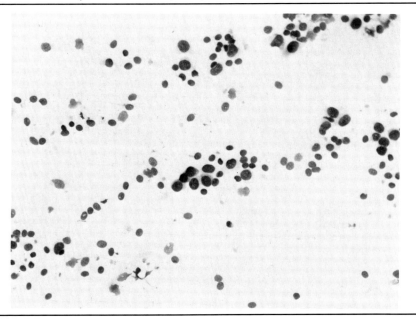

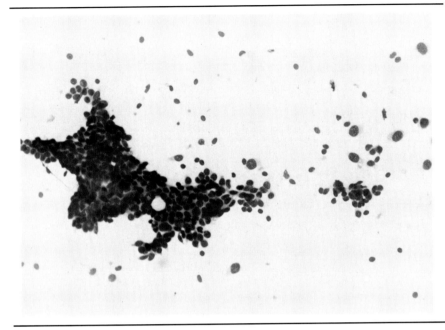

Figure 9.7.
Atypical ductal hyperplasia. Irregular cluster of ductal cells and loose atypical cells
(×200).

Figure 9.8.
Atypical ductal hyperplasia. Clump of ductal epithelial cells with blunt branching. Notice
loose enlarged nuclei (×400).

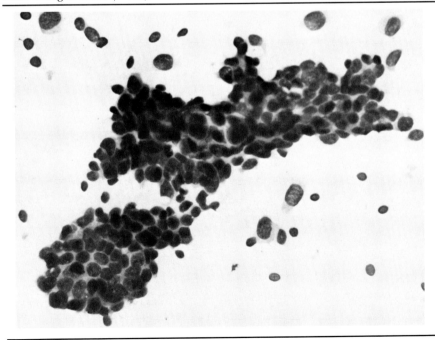

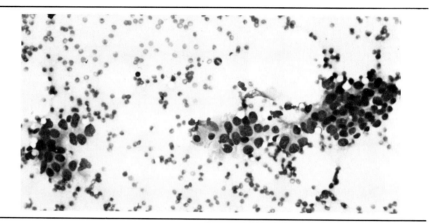

Figure 9.9.
Atypical ductal hyperplasia. Two clumps of ductal cells with moderate variation in nuclear size (×200).

Figure 9.10.
Atypical ductal hyperplasia. One of the clumps shown in Figure 9.9 (×400).

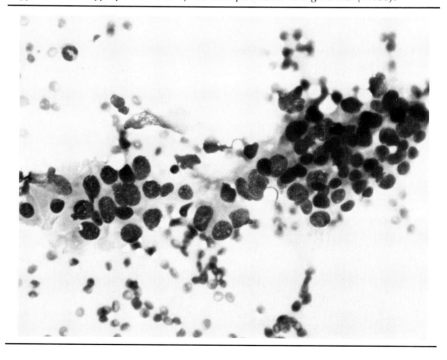

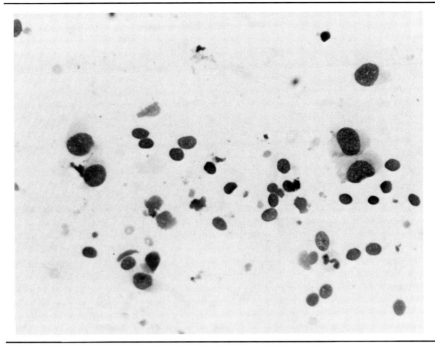

Figure 9.11.
Atypical ductal hyperplasia. Some atypical epithelial cells and many bipolar nuclei (×400).

Atypicality seen only in cell clusters (Fig. 9.10) is not as worrisome as when seen in single cells (Fig. 9.11). In these cases, we suggest an excisional biopsy (see Table 9.1).

DUCTAL HYPERPLASIA OR NEOPLASIA?

This is a particular problem when dealing with aspirates from older women. In young women, some sheets and irregular groups of cells with slightly enlarged nuclei are seen commonly in fibrocystic mastopathy. However, when observed in aspirates of postmenopausal women similar groups should raise the suspicion of a carcinoma.

When an atypical smear is obtained from a perimenopausal woman, repeat the aspiration at the time of menses. The possibility of exogenous hormones should also be investigated and brought to the referring physician's attention.

Needless to say, a positive mammogram (Lamas et al. 1984) and family history (Sattin et al. 1985) should call for more aggressive follow-up.

Table 9.1
Clinical management of ductal hyperplasia

Age	Clinical History	Palpation	Mammogram	Needle Aspiration*	Cytologic Diagnosis	What To Do
Premenopausal (20–40)	Negative	Benign**	Not done or negative	Soft or rubbery	Ductal hyperplasia	Follow-up
	Negative	Benign**	Not done or negative	Soft or rubbery	Atypical ductal hyperplasia	Repeat aspiration during menses
	Negative	Discrete mass	Negative	Rubbery	Fibroadenoma	Excise
Perimenopausal (40–50)	Negative	Benign**	Negative	Rubbery	Ductal hyperplasia	Repeat aspiration during menses, rule out exogenous hormones
	Negative	Benign**	Negative	Rubbery	Atypical ductal hyperplasia	Close follow-up or excise
Postmenopausal (50 and over)	Negative	Ill-defined, firm mass	Negative	Soft	Fat necrosis	Wait two to three weeks, excise if it does not resolve
	Negative	Benign**	Negative	Soft or firm	Atypical ductal hyperplasia versus lobular carcinoma	Excisional biopsy

*Needle aspiration: Indicates how the lesion feels when the needle is inserted.

**Benign: Lesion is multinodular, or an ill-defined thickening, or discrete and soft, or rubbery, movable, *etc.*

ATYPICAL DUCTAL HYPERPLASIA OR NEOPLASIA?

The differential diagnosis lies between atypical ductal hyperplasia and ductal adenocarcinoma when the smears are very cellular and the clumps of cells show moderate to marked variation in nuclear size, some prominent nucleoli, and some atypical single cells. If the smears consist of tightly cohesive sheets and clumps of epithelial cells with some variation in nuclear size and a few atypical single cells, we diagnose it as atypical ductal hyperplasia. In this case it is an advantage for the pathologist to have performed the aspiration. If the lesion was gritty on aspiration, this would be highly suspicious for carcinoma. The non-diagnostic smear would indicate that the malignant focus was not accurately sampled and that the patient should be reaspirated in order to obtain adequate material for a more definite diagnosis. If this is not possible (patient has developed a hematoma, *etc.*), request an excisional biopsy.

If the lesion was ill-defined and rubbery on aspiration, and the pathologist obtained multiple and generous samples, than a diagnosis of atypical ductal hyperplasia is reasonable, and the patient should be followed at frequent and regular intervals. In cases of this type, it is helpful to review again the clinical history and the results of mammograms. If either one is positive, the lesion should be excised. Dupont and Page (1985) and Page et al. (1985) have called attention to the increased risk of breast cancer in patients with atypical hyperplasia and a positive family history.

If the smears show many sheets and clusters of pleomorphic cells, with or without visible nucleoli, along with many atypical single cells, they are diagnostic of carcinoma. This is so, regardless of age, and regardless of "feeling benign on palpation," even if the mammogram is negative and there is no family history of carcinoma.

At our institution some mastectomies are performed without a frozen section, based only on a cytologic diagnosis. Hence, we approach an aspirate as we would a frozen section. If we are absolutely sure that we are dealing with a malignancy, we say so. If we have any doubt, we communicate that doubt in our written report to the clinician or surgeon, and additional diagnostic procedures are attempted.

General Diagnostic Criteria of Malignancy

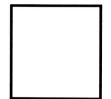
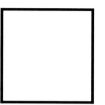

10

Exfoliative cytology recognizes that malignant cells differ from normal cells in a variety of ways. Although no single change is pathognomonic, the spectrum of changes taken together can be a reliable indicator of malignancy. This also is true of aspiration cytology; however, most criteria have been developed from Papanicolaou-stained material. Criteria are simpler for smears stained with hematologic stains.

1. The most important diagnostic criterion of malignancy is the presence of "tumor cellularity." By this we mean extremely cellular smears (Figs. 10.1 and 10.2). This is to be expected from the loss of cellular cohesiveness in malignancy. A microscopic diagnosis of carcinoma is one made at low magnification. Higher magnification helps determine the type of carcinoma.
2. The neoplastic cells show two different arrangements: clumps (Figs. 10.3 and 10.4) or clusters of cells, and single cells or loose cells (Figs. 10.5 and 10.6; Color Plates XVI–XVIII).
3. The cells must display nuclear pleomorphism (Figs. 10.5 and 10.6; Color Plates XIX and XX).

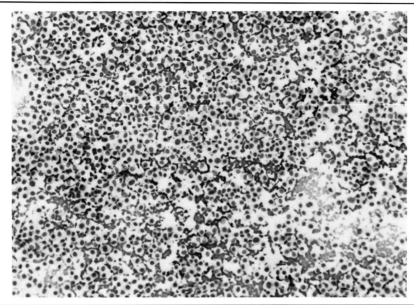

Figure 10.1.
Ductal adenocarcinoma: tumor cellularity. Innumerable loosely cohesive epithelial cells cover the entire field. Even at this low magnification one can observe the variation in nuclear size (×100). Compare with smears of fibroadenoma (Figs. 8.32 and 8.34) and fibrocystic disease (Fig. 6.9 A and B) at the same magnification.

Figure 10.2.
Ductal adenocarcinoma. Epithelial cells with some variation in nuclear size, occasional nucleoli, and delicate cytoplasm (×400).

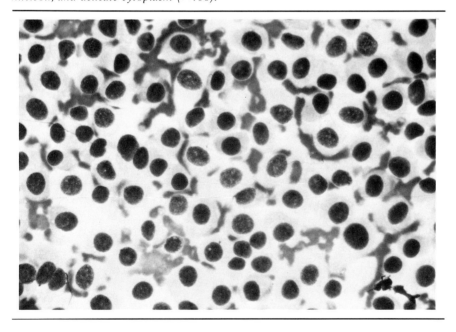

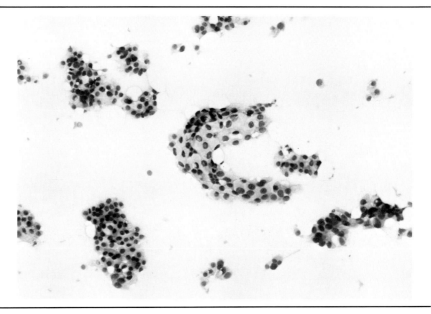

Figure 10.3.
Ductal adenocarcinoma. Neoplastic cells showing two different arrangements: clusters and sheets and a few loose cells in the background (×100).

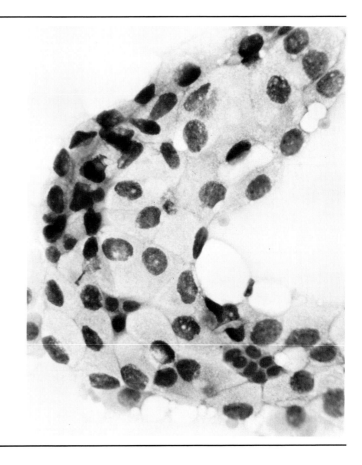

Figure 10.4.
Ductal adenocarcinoma. Higher magnification of sheet shown in Figure 10.3. Notice variation in nuclear size, well-demarcated cell borders, and glandular lumina (×400).

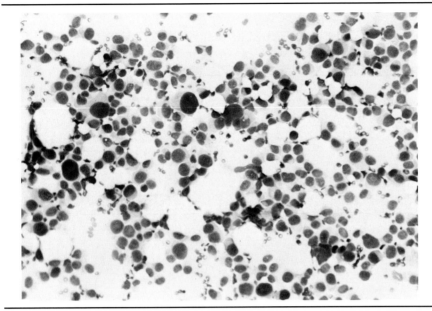

Figure 10.5.
Ductal adenocarcinoma. Sheet of loosely cohesive neoplastic cells with marked variation in nuclear size. Note the nuclear molding around glandular lumina (×200).

Figure 10.6.
Ductal adenocarcinoma. Loose epithelial cells of neoplastic nature showing marked nuclear pleomorphism. Compare the size of the nuclei with the size of the erythrocytes seen in the background (×400).

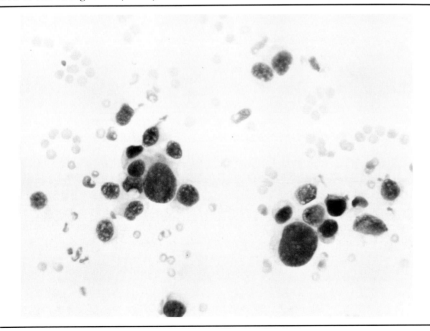

INFILTRATION

Infiltration cannot be appreciated in aspirates. Excisional biopsy remains the method of choice for studying this important criterion of malignancy. Hence, we do not make a specific diagnosis of "infiltrating adenocarcinoma." We have to assume that if the lesion is palpable it is infiltrating. Fine needle aspiration is also of no value in distinguishing early infiltration (microinvasion).

NUCLEUS

The increased size and irregularities of shape exhibited by neoplastic nuclei are well known (Color Plates XVI–XX). Thus, it is essential to remember the shape and size of the nuclei of normal ductal cells to serve as a baseline (see Figs. 6.5 and 6.6; Color Plate I). However, the nuclei of both adenoid cystic and lobular carcinomas are small and may show little or no irregularity. On the other hand, one sometimes finds enlarged, irregular nuclei in normal tissues or in fibroadenomas. Such exceptions illustrate how important it is to recognize the normal and the need to constantly exercise good judgment.

The well-known alterations in the structure of the nuclear chromatin, parachromatin, and nuclear membrane are seen only in Papanicolaou-stained material (Frost 1969). They are not observed in air-dried smears stained with Diff-Quik.

INTRANUCLEAR INCLUSIONS OR VACUOLES

Although intranuclear inclusions (vacuoles) are particularly helpful in the diagnosis of papillary carcinoma of the thyroid, they also can be observed in fibrocystic disease and in some benign and malignant mammary neoplasms. They are not generally useful as diagnostic criteria in the breast.

NUCLEOLUS

When smears are stained with Papanicolaou's technique, nucleolar alterations are some of the most constant and diagnostically important features: increase in size of nucleolus, increase in number of nucleoli, and variations in the size and shape of the nucleolus (Frost 1969). With Diff-Quik-stained material the nucleoli are not particularly evident. They are visible in some benign conditions (apocrine metaplastic cells, ductal cells with lactational changes, etc.) and are relatively conspicuous in medullary carcinoma of the breast, in poorly differentiated adenocarcinomas, and in metastatic melanomas.

INTRACELLULAR OR INTRACYTOPLASMIC LUMINA

Observed as well-demarcated intracytoplasmic spaces, intracellular or intra-cytoplasmic lumina are seen more commonly in malignant entities (Figs. 10.7 and 10.8). Rare examples have been described in adenomas. Glandular lumina or intercellular lumina are also common findings (Fig. 10.8).

Figure 10.7.
Ductal adenocarcinoma. Intracellular or intracytoplasmic lumina. Sheet of neoplastic cells, a few with a large thick-rimmed cytoplasmic vacuole, and what appears to be condensation of mucoid material in its center. Other cells show multiple small cytoplasmic vacuoles (×400).

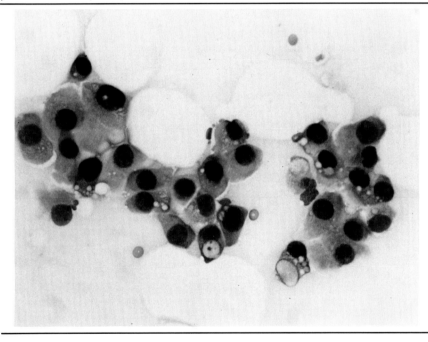

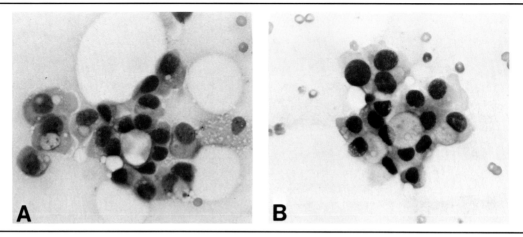

Figure 10.8.
Ductal adenocarcinoma. A glandular or intercellular lumen is seen in the center and, to the side of it, a cell with an intracytoplasmic lumen (×400).

Figure 10.9.
Long, narrow blood vessel. Notice neoplastic cells in the background (×100).

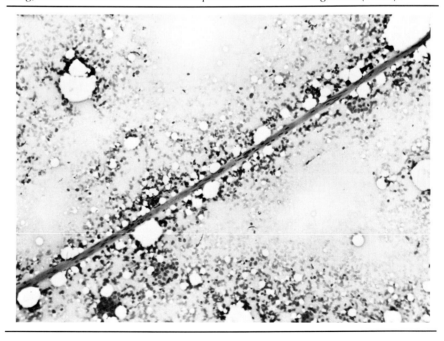

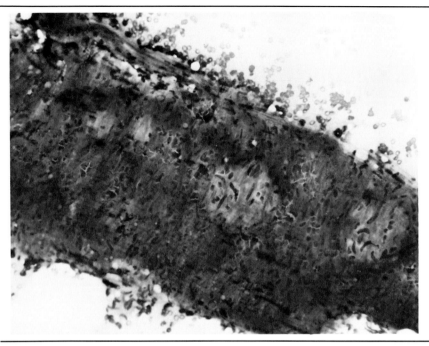

Figure 10.10.
Fragment of thicker blood vessel than in Figure 10.9, from a smear of ductal carcinoma (×200).

MITOTIC FIGURES

Mitoses indicate active growth but are not pathognomonic of malignancy. They are observed infrequently in primary breast carcinomas except in medullary carcinoma, particularly the atypical variant. Mitoses are conspicuous in metastatic melanomas (Figs. 13.1–13.3)

BLOOD VESSELS

Blood vessels are frequently found in smears of carcinomas. They may be seen as extremely long tubular structures traversing one or two low power fields (Fig. 10.9), or as shorter but thicker fragments of arterioles or veins with easily visualized muscular walls (Fig. 10.10). We would like to emphasize that capillaries are frequently seen in normal adipose tissue as well. However, if thick-walled blood vessels are seen in the fat, we become concerned that an adjacent carcinoma has not been adequately sampled. Likewise, when we see many fragments of blood vessels in smears lacking cellular atypia it becomes necessary to rule out a tubular, lobular, or a well-differentiated adenocarcinoma.

Adenocarcinomas 11

The following are cytologic criteria that we developed from a previous review of our material (Oertel and Galblum 1983). They have been tested prospectively, and modified, and to some degree expanded. However, as surgical pathologists we know that breast cancer is a heterogeneous disease (Rosen 1979b) and difficult to classify as to type because of limited sampling and the coexistence of different tumor types in the same lesion (Gallager 1984, p. 625; Rosen et al. 1972, p. 838).

DUCTAL ADENOCARCINOMAS

"Infiltrating" Ductal Carcinoma

On physical examination the lesion may display the clinical characteristics of malignancy, that is, a single or dominant firm mass fixed to the overlying skin, skin dimpling and nipple retraction, and edema of the overlying skin (peau d'orange). When introducing the needle, a gritty consistency will be felt. These lesions bleed easily on aspiration. Thus, one should be careful not to produce a hematoma. Make sure to apply pressure on the area after performing the aspiration. If some extravasation can be seen, place an ice cube wrapped in plastic on the site for a few minutes.

The smears are extremely cellular (tumor cellularity) (Figs. 10.1 and 10.2). There are many cellular clusters of different sizes and degrees of cohesiveness (Color Plates XVI–XVIII) and large numbers of isolated epithelial cells. Marked nuclear atypia should be observed both in the cellular clusters and in the isolated cells (Figs. 10.3–10.6). There is a high nuclear/cytoplasmic ratio; the nuclei are large and vary in size and shape (Color Plates XIX and XX). Some bizarre nuclei are evident. Mitotic figures are uncommon and this is a discrepancy with the histologic findings, for which we have no good explanation.

Carcinoma with Necrosis (Comedocarcinoma)

In these cases, the smears generally are fairly thick and the aspirated material is difficult to smear. There is abundant necrotic amorphous debris, and in it many clusters and single atypical cells are observed (Figs. 11.1 and 11.2). As a rule inflammatory cells are not very numerous.

In other areas where there is less necrotic debris and the cellular characteristics can be observed more readily, nuclear pleomorphism is quite evident (Fig. 11.3). Many of the cellular clumps have irregular shapes and show superimposition of the cells and varying degrees of cohesiveness. The cytoplasm is conspicuous and varies in density and degree of preservation. Intercellular and intracytoplasmic lumina are easily observed. Occasional nucleoli are seen. Bizarre cells are fairly common (Fig. 11.4).

Figure 11.1.
Comedocarcinoma. A few small groups and some isolated neoplastic cells are seen in a necrotic background (×100).

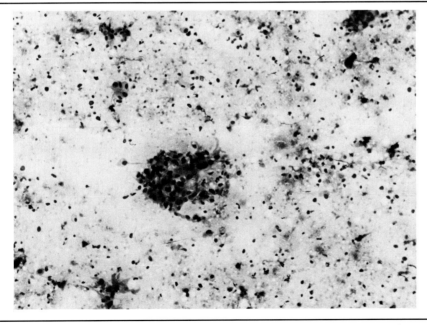

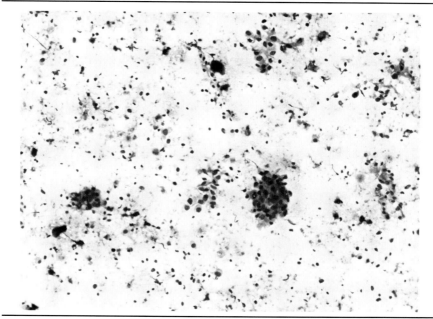

Figure 11.2.
Comedocarcinoma. Even at this low magnification the nuclear pleomorphism is evident in the central cells. Necrotic debris lies in the background (×100).

Figure 11.3.
Comedocarcinoma. We have chosen a field with very little necrosis in order to demonstrate the nuclear pleomorphism in these cellular clusters (×200).

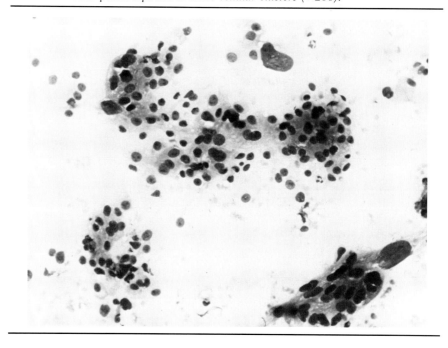

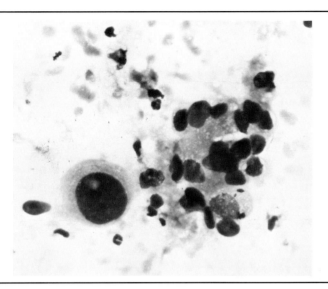

Figure 11.4.
Comedocarcinoma. Group of neoplastic cells, one quite bizarre (×400).

Papillary Carcinoma

The few lesions that we have aspirated have always been hemorrhagic. Aspiration produces dark brown, thick fluid resembling chocolate syrup. The smears are extremely cellular (tumor cellularity). In our experience this lesion frequently yields large fragments of tissue. In addition, the most striking finding is the presence of a dense fibrous core in the largest fragments of tissue (Fig. 11.5). The epithelial cells are moderately enlarged and have well-defined cytoplasm and regular nuclei (Figs. 11.6 and 11.7). Some intracellular lumina are seen.

Colloid Carcinoma

On aspiration the lesion is soft, and abundant mucoid material is obtained. This is quite evident when contents of the needle hub are squirted onto the glass slides. The smears are thick. At low magnification there is abundant pale pink or bluish-pink mucin (Figs. 11.8 and 11.9; Color Plates XXI and XXII). Large numbers of cells, singly and in tight groups, frequently are present (Fig. 11.10). Sometimes there are only a few cells and the sample consists mostly of mucus. At low magnification a conspicuous feature is the presence of many branching blood vessels traversing the pools of mucus (Figs. 11.8, 11.9, and 11.11). With higher magnification many loosely cohesive epithelial cells with a moderate amount of cytoplasm and round nuclei are visible (Figs. 11.10–11.13). In some

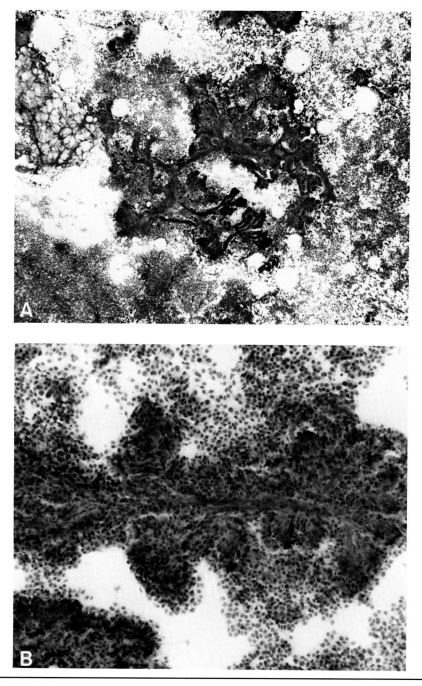

Figure 11.5.
Papillary carcinoma. Large fragment of tissue with a central fibrovascular core and fingerlike projections extruding from it. A. (×40). B. (×100).

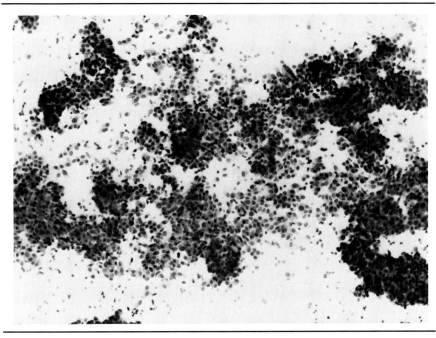

Figure 11.6.
Papillary carcinoma. Large irregular groups of epithelial cells, devoid of a fibrovascular core. They show variable degrees of cohesiveness (×100).

Figure 11.7.
Papillary carcinoma. At higher magnification the nuclei are regular. However, notice that the neoplastic nuclei are at least two to three times the size of the red blood cells in the background (×400).

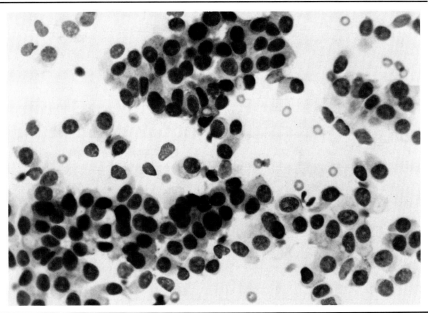

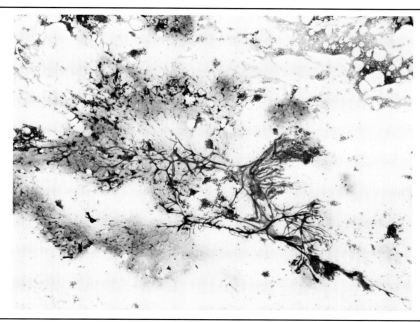

Figure 11.8.
Colloid carcinoma. Abundant mucoid material and a few groups of barely discernible neoplastic epithelial cells. The complex branching structure corresponds to numerous capillaries that are one of the hallmarks of this entity (×40).

Figure 11.9.
Colloid carcinoma. Higher magnification of Figure 11.8. Neoplastic epithelial cells surrounded by profusely branching capillaries and mucoid material at the edges of the picture (×100).

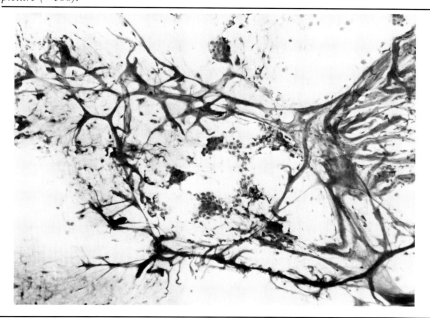

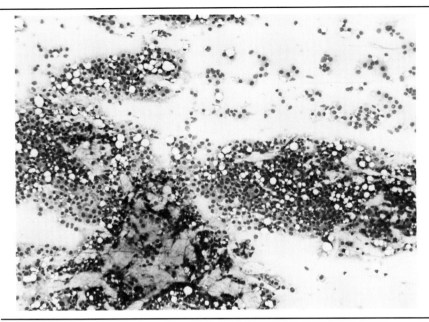

Figure 11.10.
Colloid carcinoma: tumor cellularity. Notice scant mucoid material in the lower left hand corner and large numbers of epithelial cells (×100).

Figure 11.11.
Colloid carcinoma. Thin mucoid material and a vacuolated background, large numbers of epithelial cells with barely discernible cytoplasm, and a branching capillary with plump endothelial cells (×200).

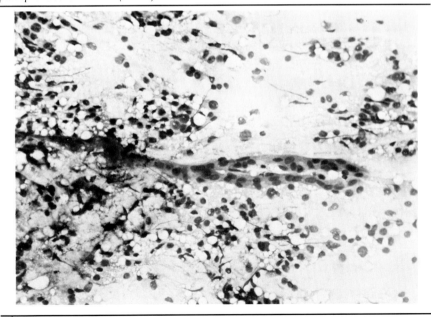

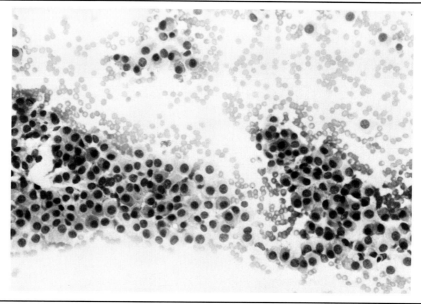

Figure 11.12.
Colloid carcinoma: tumor cellularity. In this photograph the relatively small neoplastic cells are the predominant element. However, when compared to the red blood cells one can appreciate that their nuclei are at least twice the size of the erythrocytes (×200).

Figure 11.13.
Colloid carcinoma. Notice the delicate to coarse cytoplasmic vacuolation and the variation in nuclear size (×400). Binucleated cell in the inset (×400).

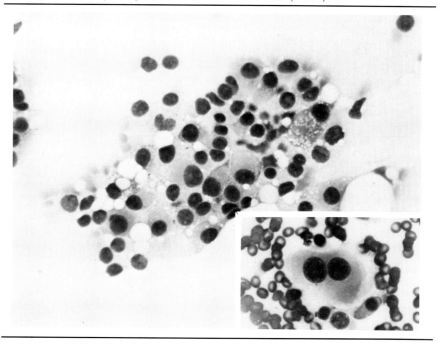

cases the nuclei are regular, while in others the nuclear size varies. Some nucleoli sometimes can be seen. Cytoplasmic vacuoles of different sizes are frequently evident. The cells in clusters display similar cytologic features. The mucoid background may appear vacuolated.

These lesions also bleed easily, and most of the smears show abundant blood (from recent hemorrhage) mixed with the mucus.

Medullary Carcinoma

When aspirated, medullary carcinoma is soft and bleeds easily. In some instances the smears show predominantly lymphoid tissue and a few small groups of atypical epithelial cells (Fig. 11.14). Sometimes one has to search for the cellular clusters that will indicate an epithelial lesion rather than a lymphoma. Other cases exhibit tumor cellularity (Fig. 11.15) with numerous large thick clumps of malignant epithelial cells surrounded by many lymphoid and plasma cells. In some other cases irregular naked nuclei with prominent nucleoli are the most conspicuous characteristic (Figs. 11.16 – 11.18; Color Plate XXIII). Sometimes abnormal mitoses are present (Color Plate XXIV).

Many lymphocytes as well as some histiocytes and plasma cells are observed (Fig. 11.19). The background of the smears is usually proteinaceous or hemorrhagic. Occasionally one can find areas of necrosis.

Figure 11.14.
Medullary carcinoma. In this particular case the lymphoid tissue predominates, and there are very few small groups of epithelial cells (×100).

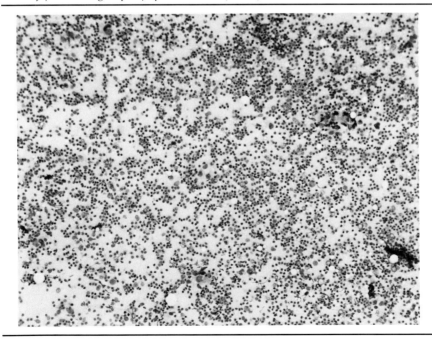

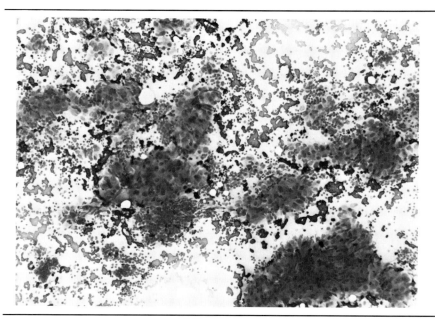

Figure 11.15.
Medullary carcinoma. Another case in which the neoplastic cells form large, thick, irregular clumps. Notice the lymphocytes and red blood cells in the background (×100).

Figure 11.16.
Medullary carcinoma. The neoplastic cells in this smear show lack of cohesiveness and inconspicuous cytoplasm. Cases like this can be confused with malignant lymphoma (×200).

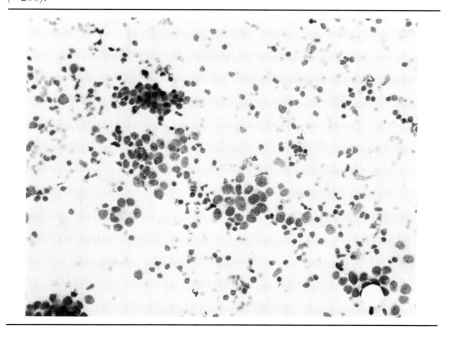

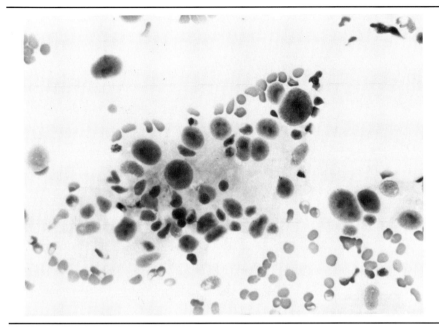

Figure 11.17.
Medullary carcinoma. Neoplastic cells with prominent nucleoli. The small hyperchromatic nuclei correspond to lymphocytes (×400).

Figure 11.18.
Medullary carcinoma. Some loosely cohesive epithelial cells with vacuolated cytoplasm (×400).

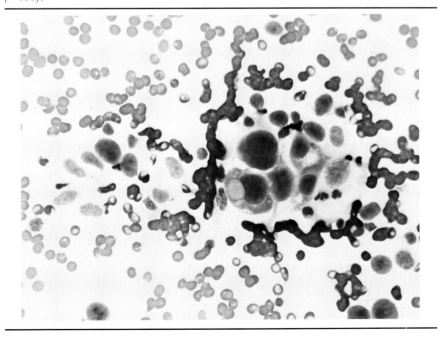

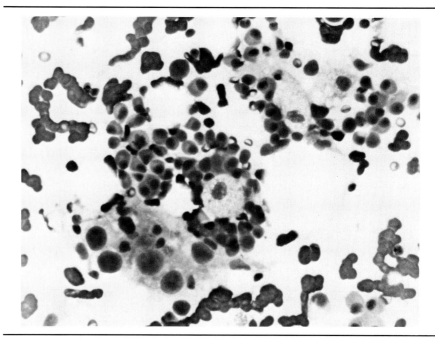

Figure 11.19.
Medullary carcinoma. A few neoplastic cells, some foamy histiocytes, and many plasma cells (×400).

RELATIVELY RARE DUCTAL CARCINOMAS

Apocrine Carcinoma

Smears from apocrine carcinoma are characterized by tumor cellularity and an inflammatory background consisting of blood, polymorphonuclear leukocytes, some foamy histiocytes, and occasional multinucleated histiocytes. Most of the malignant epithelial cells appear in large clusters or cords (Figs. 11.20 and 11.21), and they are reminiscent of the apocrine ductal cells of fibrocystic disease (Color Plates XXV and XXVI). Some have delicate cytoplasm but the majority have dense cytoplasm with "apocrine snouts" and basophilia of the cell borders. Cytoplasmic granules are seen frequently. They vary in size and color, from grayish blue to red. Because of the marked variation in nuclear size they are recognized as malignant (Figs. 11.22 and 11.23). Although irregular and multiple nucleoli are seen, the nucleoli are not as prominent as in medullary carcinoma. Atypical naked nuclei, loose cells, and small groups of cells are also present. Microcalcifications are seen often (Figs. 11.20 and 11.21). Occasionally the pathologist cannot distinguish this carcinoma from an exuberant apocrine metaplasia in fibrocystic disease. Therefore, when in doubt, remember to request an excisional biopsy.

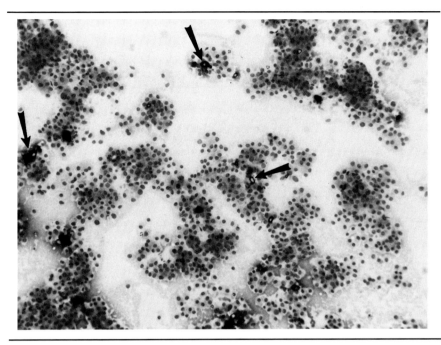

Figure 11.20.
Apocrine carcinoma: tumor cellularity. The neoplastic cells are arranged in cords. Notice microcalcifications (arrows) *(×100).*

Figure 11.21.
Apocrine carcinoma. Cords of neoplastic cells and numerous microcalcifications are seen (×200).

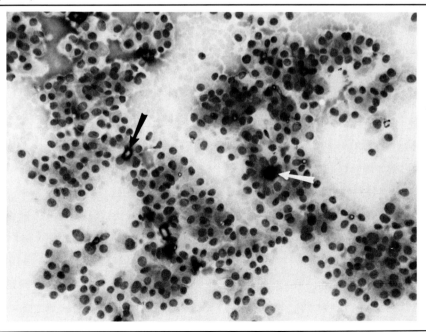

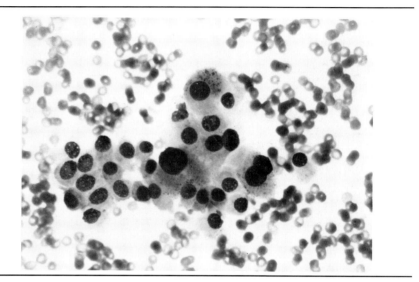

Figure 11.22.
Apocrine carcinoma. Notice the resemblance to apocrine metaplastic cells (compare with Fig. 6.9). The neoplastic cells show more variation in nuclear size (×400).

Figure 11.23.
Apocrine carcinoma. Sheet of neoplastic cells with variable nuclear sizes. Note single cell in left upper corner (×400).

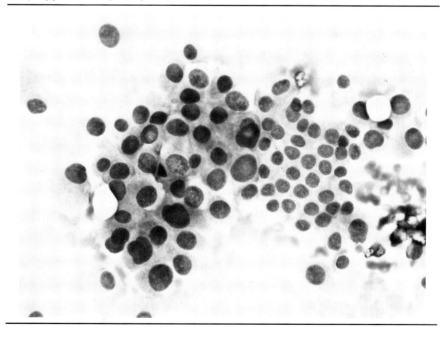

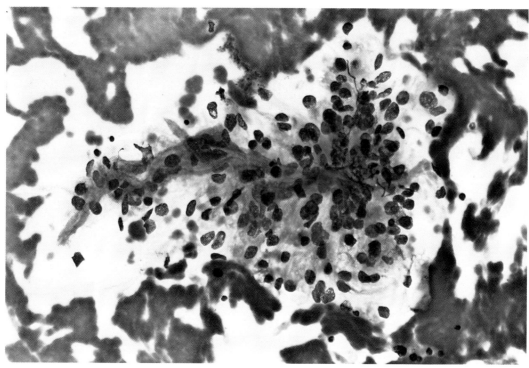

Color Plate XXXI.
Metastatic renal cell carcinoma. Cluster of cells with a pink fibrovascular core (×320).

Color Plate XXXII.
Schwannoma or neurilemoma. Very cellular tissue fragment with "palisading" ovoid nuclei (×320).

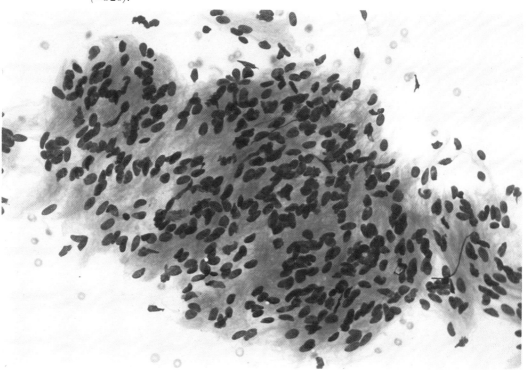

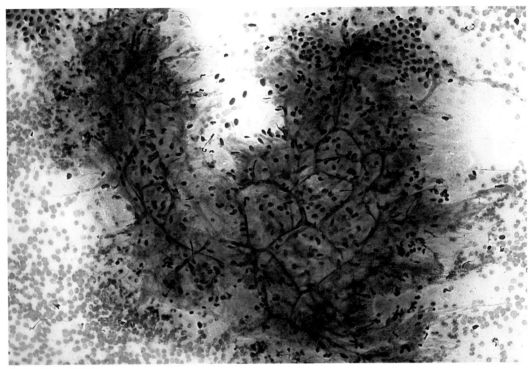

Color Plate XXIX.
Cystosarcoma phyllodes. Large fragment of fibrous connective tissue and group of ductal cells (×160). Compare with fibroadenoma, Color Plate XII, at same magnification.

Color Plate XXX.
Cystosarcoma phyllodes. Fibrous connective tissue traversed by branching capillaries (×320). Compare with Color Plate XIII.

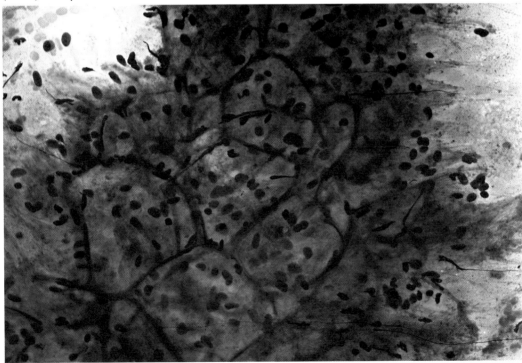

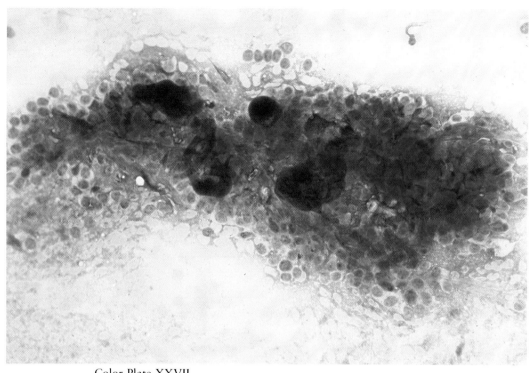

Color Plate XXVII.
Adenoid cystic carcinoma. Tissue fragment with bright pink globules (×320).

Color Plate XXVIII.
Adenoid cystic carcinoma. Bright pink, dense mucoid material forming "globules" and tubular structures (×320).

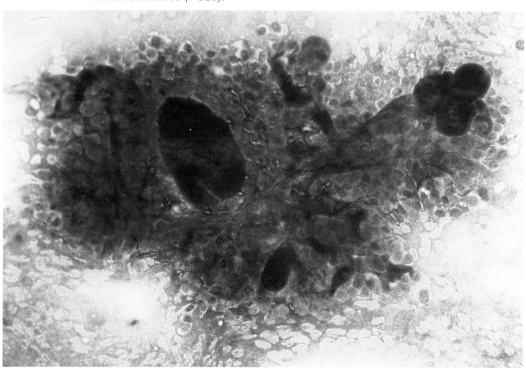

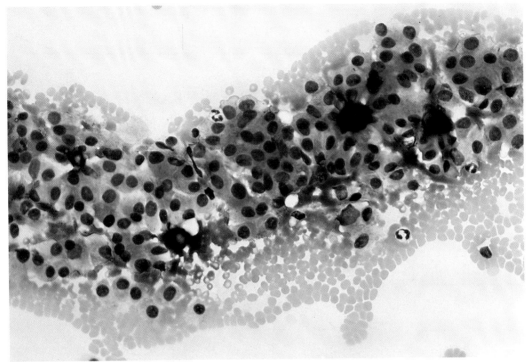

Color Plate XXV.
Apocrine carcinoma. Neoplastic cells and numerous microcalcifications (×320).

Color Plate XXVI.
Apocrine carcinoma. Neoplastic cells show variation in nuclear size and some prominent nucleoli (×640).

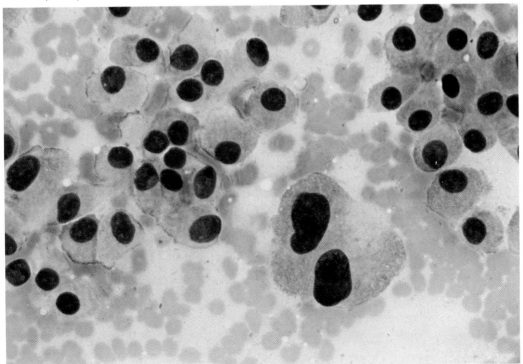

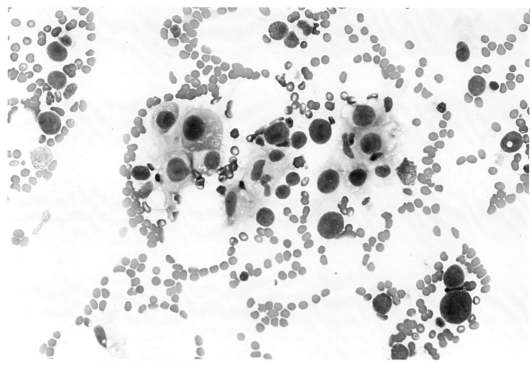

Color Plate XXIII.
Medullary carcinoma. Some neoplastic cells with delicate cytoplasm and others devoid of it (naked nuclei of variable size) show prominent nucleoli (x320).

Color Plate XXIV.
Atypical medullary carcinoma. Abnormal mitotic figure is apparent (×640).

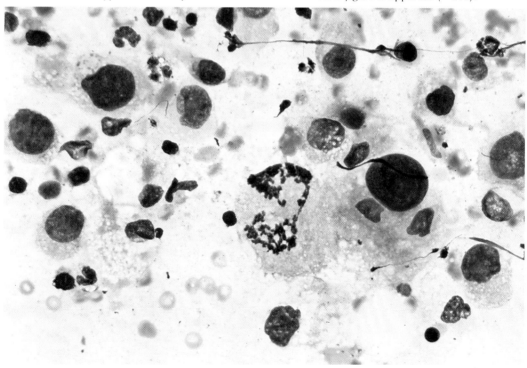

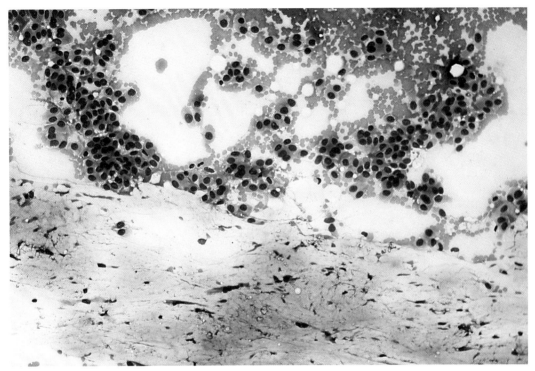

Color Plate XXI.
Colloid carcinoma. Mucoid material and groups of neoplastic cells (×160).

Color Plate XXII.
Colloid carcinoma. Very cellular smear, "tumor cellularity," and arborescent blood vessels in a pale mucous pool (×160).

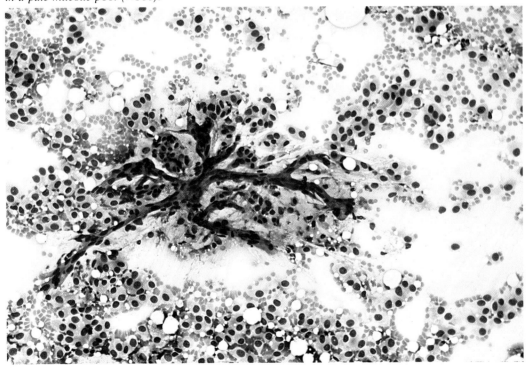

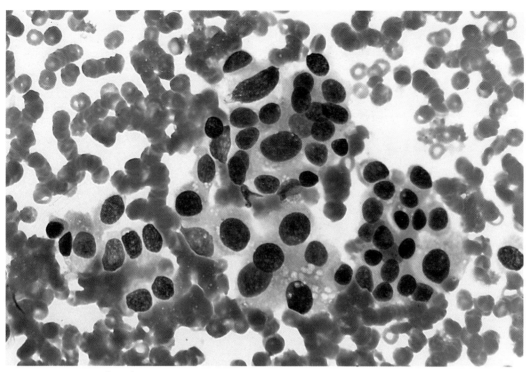

Color Plate XIX.
Ductal adenocarcinoma. These cells show moderate variation in nuclear size (×640). Compare with benign ductal cells (Color Plate I) at the same magnification.

Color Plate XX.
Ductal adenocarcinoma. Large and markedly atypical ductal cells (×640). Compare with cells in Color Plate XIX, from another case of ductal adenocarcinoma, at the same magnification.

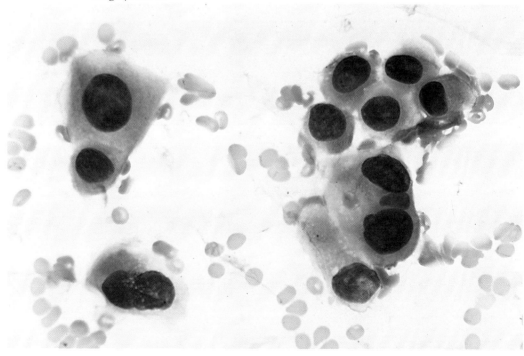

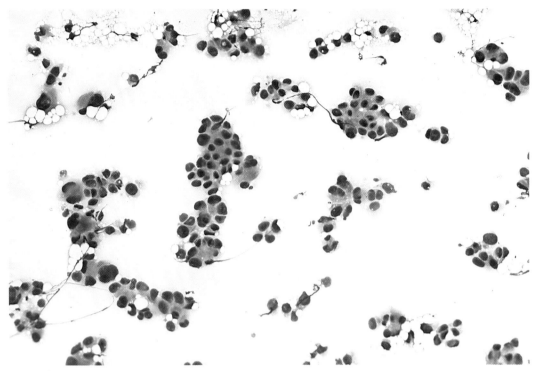

Color Plate XVII.
Ductal adenocarcinoma. Smaller clusters of atypical cells. The cellular atypia is evident even at this low magnification (×160).

Color Plate XVIII.
Ductal adenocarcinoma. Loosely cohesive cells with scant and delicate cytoplasm (×320).

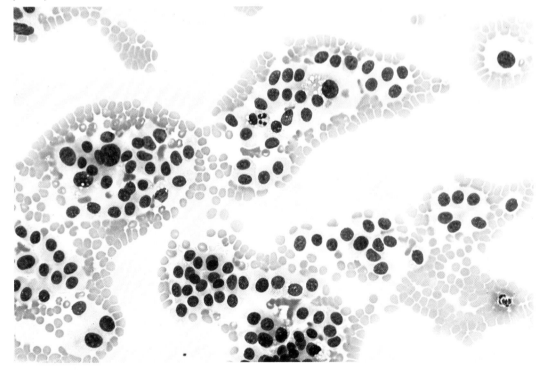

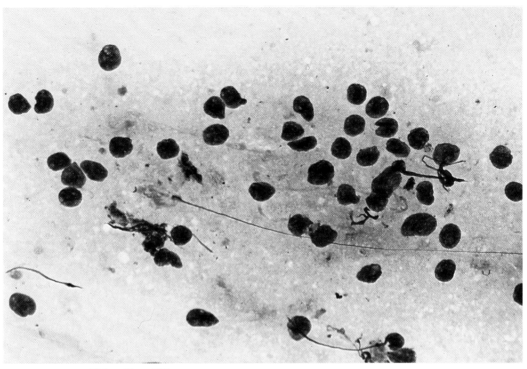

Color Plate XV.
Granular cell myoblastoma. No cellular borders are observed. Some nuclei are crushed and distorted (×640).

Color Plate XVI.
Ductal adenocarcinoma. Most of the neoplastic cells are arranged in large irregular clusters (×160). Compare with the epithelial cells seen in a fibroadenoma (Color Plate XII) at the same magnification.

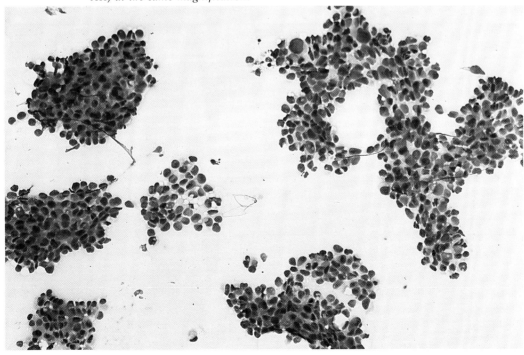

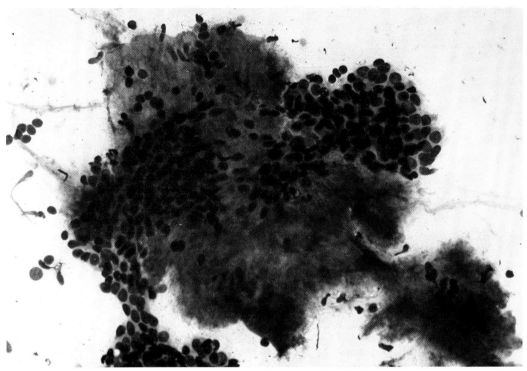

Color Plate XIII.
Fibroadenoma. Fibrous connective tissue and thick clumps of ductal cells (×320).

Color Plate XIV.
Granular cell myoblastoma. Note marked fragility of the cytoplasm and some "nuclear threads" (×160).

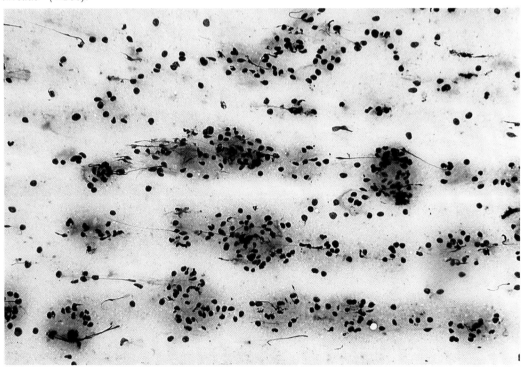

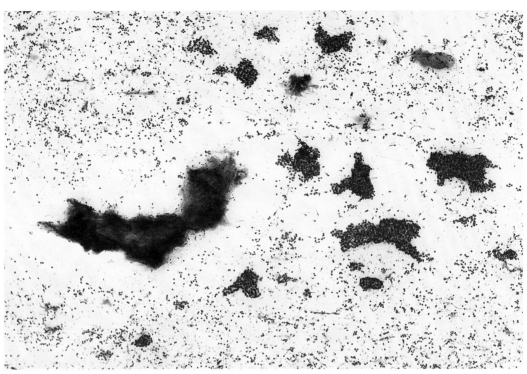

Color Plate XI.
Fibroadenoma. Very cellular smear with large fragments of connective tissue (×64).

Color Plate XII.
Fibroadenoma. Very cellular smear. Thick clumps of ductal cells, fibrous connective tissue and naked nuclei (×160).

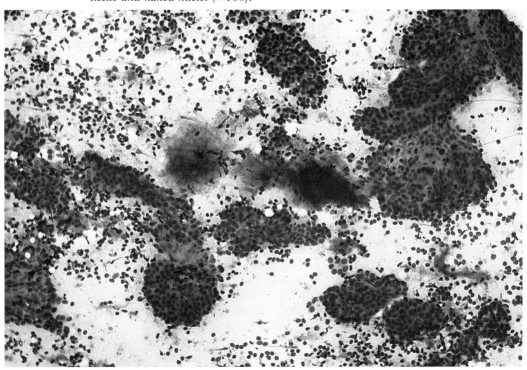

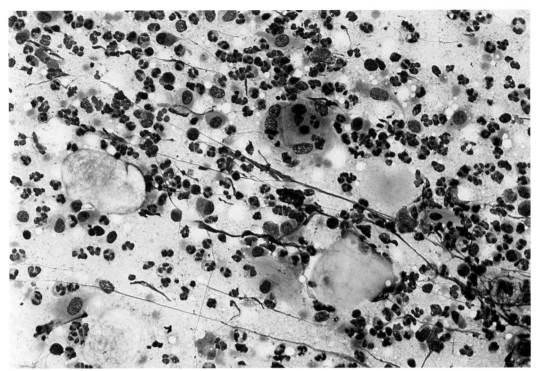

Color Plate IX.
Subareolar abscess. Anucleated squames and inflammatory cells (×320).

Color Plate X.
Granulomatous mastitis. Multinucleated histiocyte with phagocytized suture material (×640).

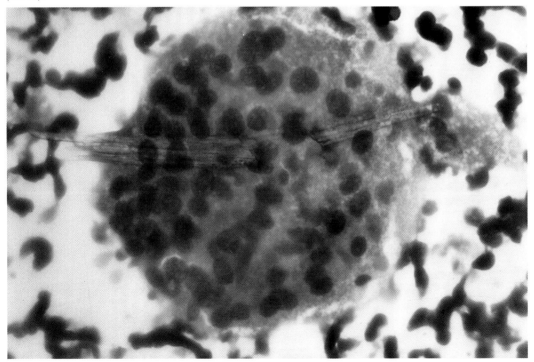

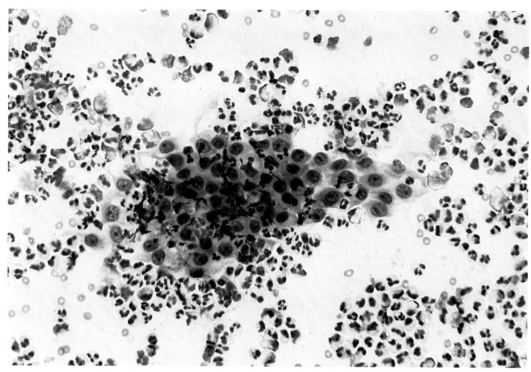

Color Plate VII.
Acute mastitis or abscess. Large cluster of atypical ductal cells surrounded by leukocytes (×320).

Color Plate VIII.
Subareolar abscess. Branching capillary, anucleated squames (pale blue and angular clear spaces), and many inflammatory cells in the background (×160).

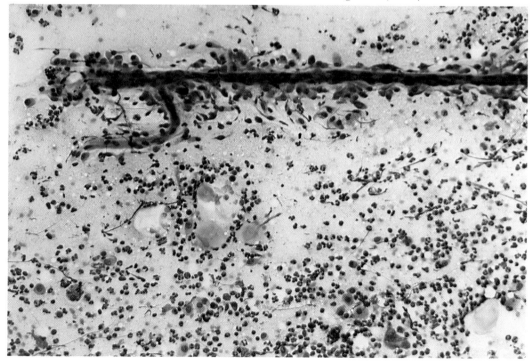

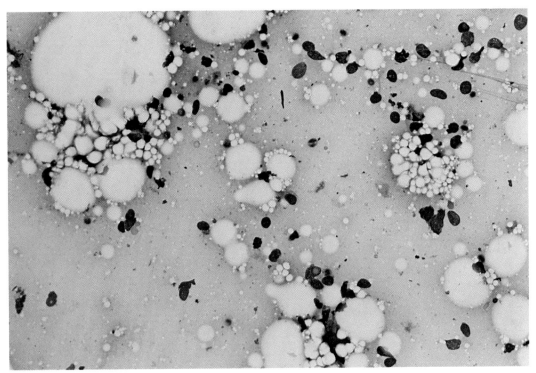

Color Plate V.
Lactation. Bubbly smear (×320).

Color Plate VI.
Lactation. Branching clump of ductal cells with prominent nucleoli. Notice "bubbly"
background (×640).

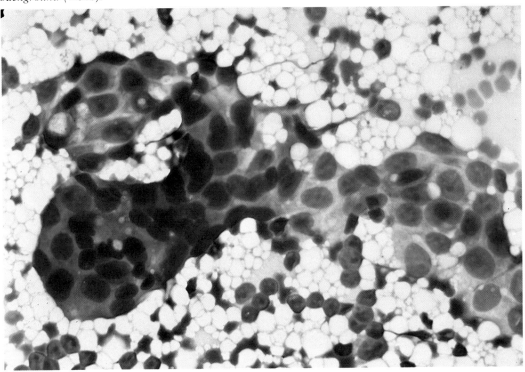

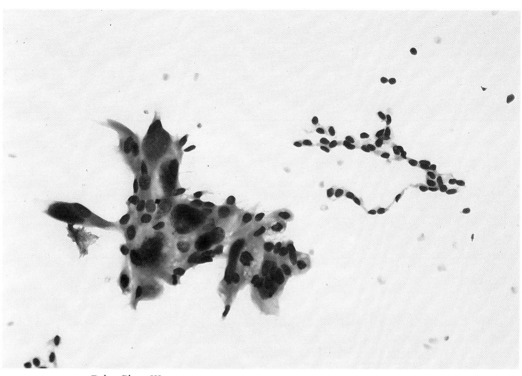

Color Plate III.
Ductal cells. Those in the larger group show squamous metaplastic changes (×320).

Color Plate IV.
Organizing hematoma. Two atypical fibroblasts (×700).

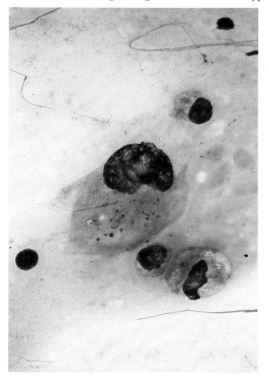

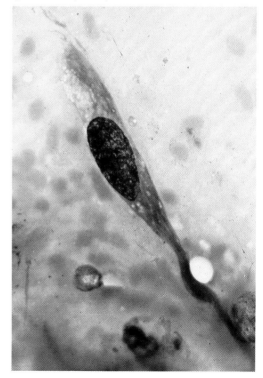

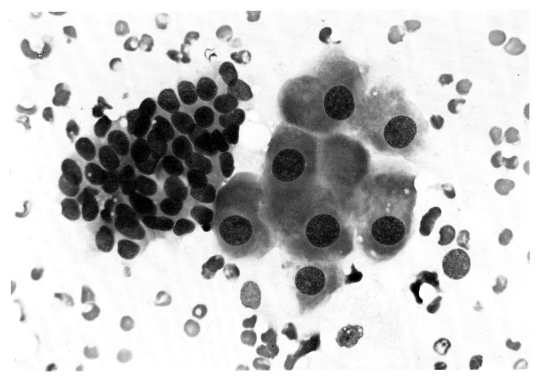

Color Plate I.
Ductal cells and apocrine metaplastic cells (×640).

Color Plate II.
Ductal cells surrounded by platelets. Many red blood cells and some leukocytes are observed in the background (×640).

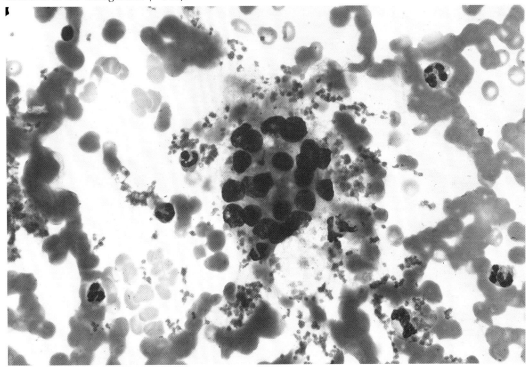

Adenoid Cystic Carcinoma

This is a relatively rare lesion but cytologically quite characteristic. The features are the same whether we are dealing with an adenoid cystic carcinoma of the breast, of the salivary glands, or of the bronchi. On aspiration, our only example was soft to palpation. The smears show large numbers of cells (Fig. 11.24) and a pale pink mucoid background in which there are bright pink dense globules (Figs. 11.25 and 11.26). At higher magnification the epithelial cells have very regular nuclei and scant cytoplasm. Occasional nucleoli are seen. The dense pink globules, most of which are surrounded by the small and fairly regular epithelial cells, are pathognomonic of this entity. Sometimes the dense pink material (on a lateral view) displays a tubular appearance (Fig. 11.27; Color Plates XXVII and XXVIII).

Tubular Carcinoma

The smears reveal tumor cellularity (Fig. 11.28) and at low magnification a pattern somewhat reminiscent of a fibroadenoma. However, on detailed examination one should notice that the groups of ductal cells resembling blunt branching (Fig. 11.29) are not as complex as those in fibroadenomas (Fig. 8.35).

Figure 11.24.
Adenoid cystic carcinoma. Large, thick, irregular tissue fragments and loose neoplastic epithelial cells: (tumor cellularity) (×100).

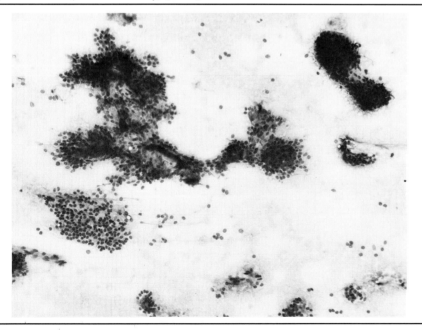

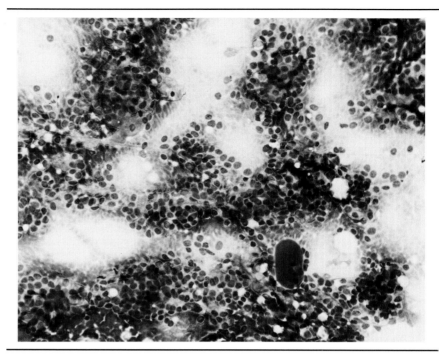

Figure 11.25.
Adenoid cystic carcinoma. Thick fragments composed of regular epithelial cells with very scant cytoplasm. Notice the dark, dense globule toward the lower part of the picture (×200).

They also have a central lumen and their configuration is that of a tubule (Figs. 11.29 and 11.30). The fibrocollagenous tissue fragments are usually small and tightly attached to cell clumps. There are no sheets of cells with a honeycomb appearance such as are seen in fibroadenoma. The groups of cells show many intercellular or glandular lumina (cribriform pattern) (Figs. 11.31 and 11.32). Intracytoplasmic lumina also are numerous and sometimes exhibit small, round, condensed mucus droplets. The nuclei are small and regular with an occasional enlarged, atypical nucleus (Fig. 11.30). The chromatin is conspicuously loose, and nucleoli are frequently seen. There are many loose cells in the background.

Inflammatory Carcinoma

Essentially this is a clinical diagnosis. The breast is enlarged, swollen, erythematous, and has extensive peau d'orange. A discrete lesion may or may not be palpated. Aspirates reveal large numbers of malignant epithelial cells both singly and in clusters (Fig. 11.33). At higher magnification the marked variation in nuclear size is evident (Figs. 11.34 and 11.35). Some cells have finely vacuolated cytoplasm (Figs. 11.35 and 11.36). Numerous polymorphonuclear leukocytes,

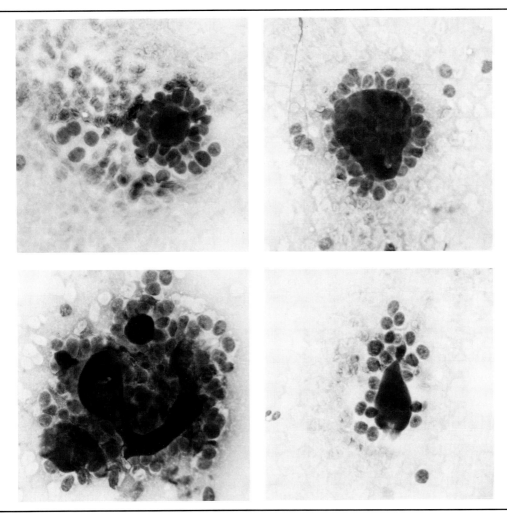

Figure 11.26.
Adenoid cystic carcinoma. This composite shows the pathognomonic "round globules" of mucoid material surrounded by the neoplastic cells. Notice the uniformity of the neoplastic nuclei (×400).

and some lymphocytes and plasma cells may be seen adjacent to the epithelial cells.

Carcinoma with Carcinoid Features

We have seen only one example. The smears are extremely cellular (Figs. 11.37–11.39), and some fields are reminiscent of lymphomas (Figs. 11.38 and 11.39). However, many small groups of cells are present (Fig. 11.37). This cellular cohesiveness betrays the epithelial nature of the lesion in contrast to malignant lymphoma (Fig. 11.40). Nuclear fragility is marked.

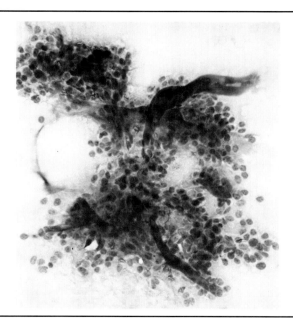

Figure 11.27.
Adenoid cystic carcinoma. Large numbers of cohesive neoplastic cells showing regular nuclei. The dense mucoid material adopts a cylindrical shape when seen on a lateral view (×200).

Figure 11.28.
Tubular carcinoma. Many groups of ductal cells, some with glandular lumina (×100).

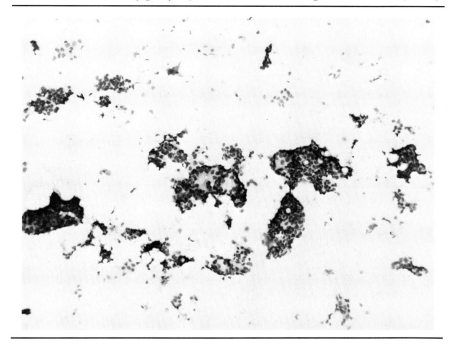

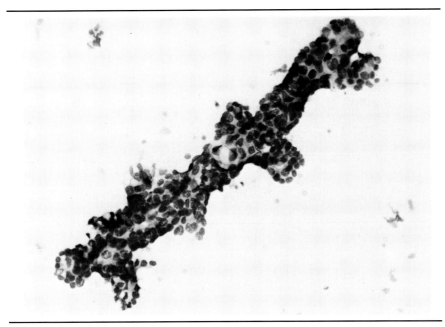

Figure 11.29.
Tubular carcinoma. Compare these small blunt projections with those of fibroadenomas (Fig. 8.35) (×200).

Figure 11.30.
Tubular carcinoma. Notice enlarged nucleus in tubular structure (arrow) *(×200).*

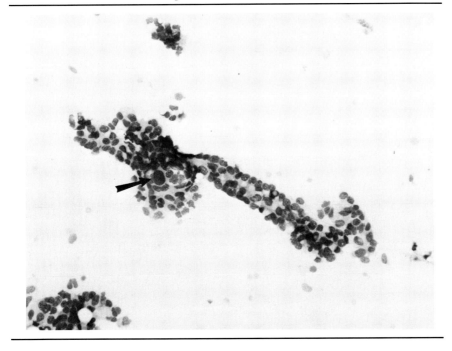

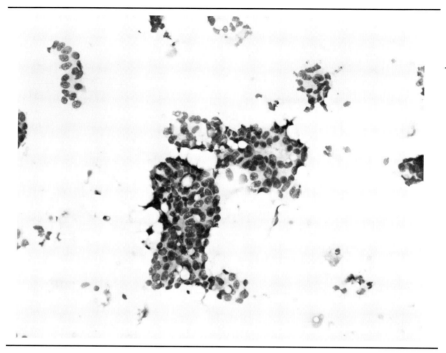

Figure 11.31.
Tubular carcinoma. Large groups of cells with multiple glandular lumina (cribriform pattern) (×200).

Figure 11.32.
Tubular carcinoma. Cribriform pattern. Notice loose chromatin in some of the nuclei (×400).

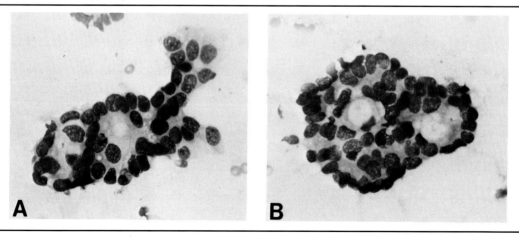

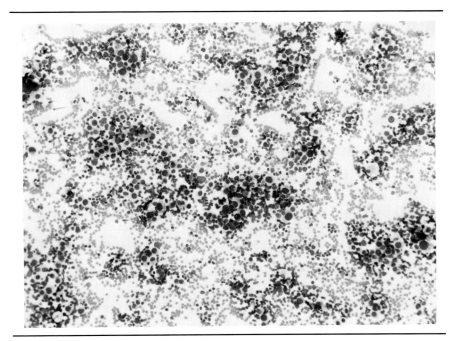

Figure 11.33.
Inflammatory carcinoma: tumor cellularity (×100).

Figure 11.34.
Inflammatory carcinoma. Notice variation in nuclear size of neoplastic cells (×200).

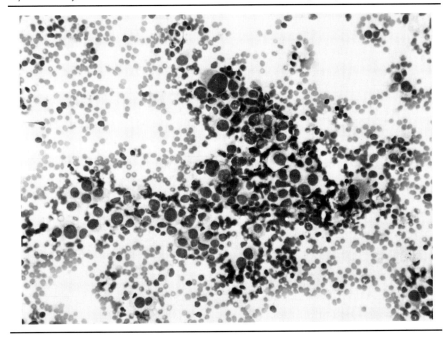

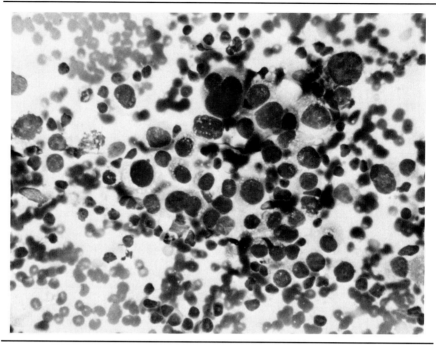

Figure 11.35.
Inflammatory carcinoma. Many erythrocytes and some leukocytes in the background.
Some of the neoplastic cells show small cytoplasmic vacuoles (×400).

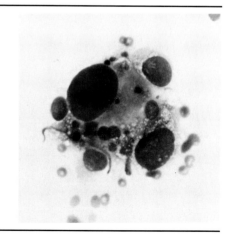

Figure 11.36.
Inflammatory carcinoma. Bizarre epithelial cells
(×400). Notice that the magnification is the same
as in Figure 11.35.

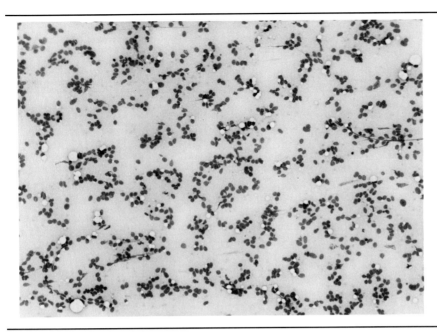

Figure 11.37.
Carcinoma with carcinoid features. Large numbers of monotonous neoplastic cells. There is a tendency to form short cords (×100).

Figure 11.38.
Carcinoma with carcinoid features (tumor cellularity). Most of the nuclei are regular, but scattered throughout the field are occasional moderately enlarged nuclei (×200).

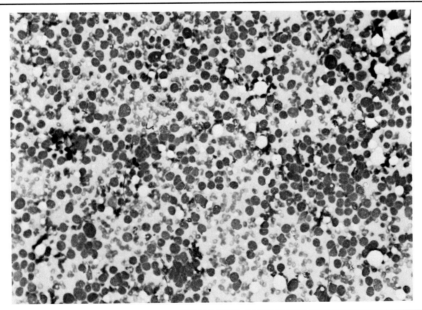

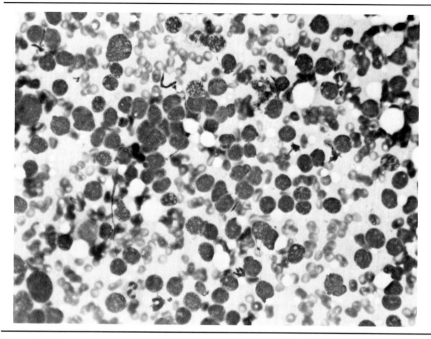

Figure 11.39.
Carcinoma with carcinoid features. Loosely cohesive neoplastic cells with regular nuclei.
Notice nuclear strands due to cellular fragility (×400).

Figure 11.40.
Carcinoma with carcinoid features. Tightly cohesive group of neoplastic nuclei showing
nuclear molding and granular chromatin (×1000).

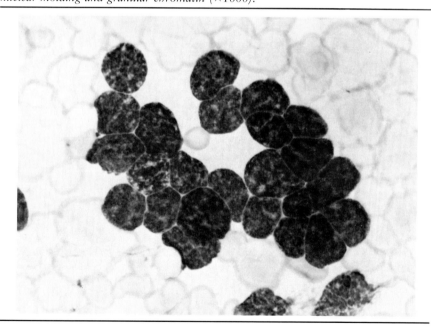

Carcinoma with Multinucleated Giant Cells

Our only case was initially aspirated by a surgeon and was not diagnostic. The patient was then referred to the pathologist. Physical examination revealed an elongated, sausage-shaped lesion as if a duct had been blocked. On aspiration the lesion felt soft.

The smears are very cellular (tumor cellularity). However, the cells are relatively small and have very regular nuclei (Figs. 11.41 and 11.42). Large numbers of multinucleated giant cells, similar to those seen in granulomatous processes are observed (Figs. 11.41, 11.43−11.45). In other areas the lesion is reminiscent of fibroadenoma (Fig. 11.42). At higher magnification occasional atypical cells are seen with enlarged bland nuclei and moderate amounts of cytoplasm (Fig. 11.44). Some microcalcifications are present (Fig. 11.46). Due to the lack of cellular pleomorphism and the presence of large numbers of multinucleated histiocytes, no definite diagnosis of malignancy was made and a surgical biopsy was recommended. Review of the histology revealed a ductal carcinoma with multinucleated giant cells (Agnantis and Rosen 1979; Pettinato et al. 1984).

Figure 11.41.
Carcinoma with multinucleated giant cells. At this low magnification we can appreciate the proteinaceous background with many naked nuclei, the tight cellular clusters, and some multinucleated giant cells (×100).

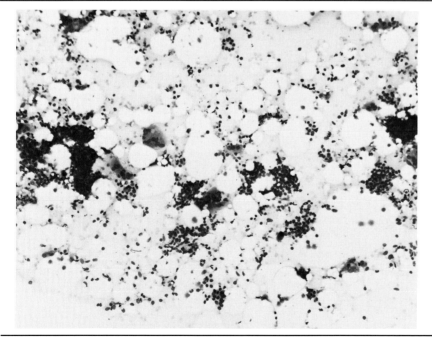

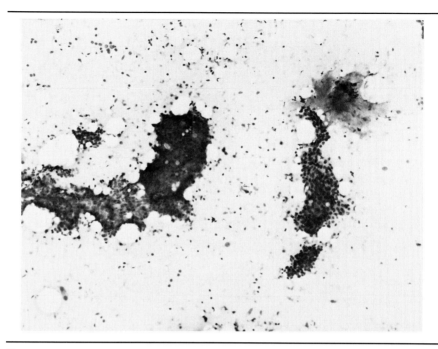

Figure 11.42.
Carcinoma with multinucleated giant cells. This particular field could be easily inter-changed with that of a fibroadenoma. Notice the fibrocollagenous tissue fragment at the upper right corner (×100).

Figure 11.43.
Carcinoma with multinucleated giant cells. Two multinucleated giant cells are seen. The adjacent cell groups show slight variation in nuclear size. A few bipolar nuclei are seen in the background (arrow) (×200).

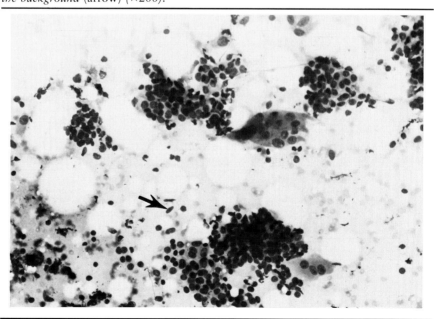

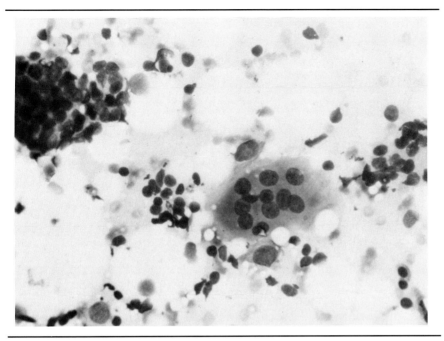

Figure 11.44.
Carcinoma with multinucleated giant cells. Adjacent to the multinucleated giant cell are two large atypical cells (×400).

Figure 11.45.
Carcinoma with multinucleated giant cells. No suggestion of atypia or malignancy in this particular field (×400).

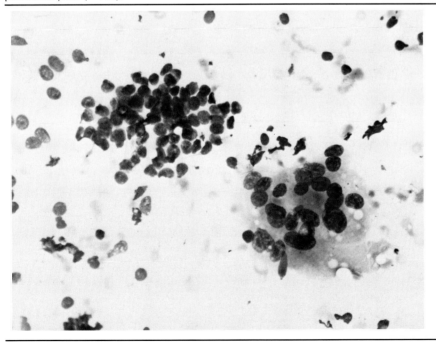

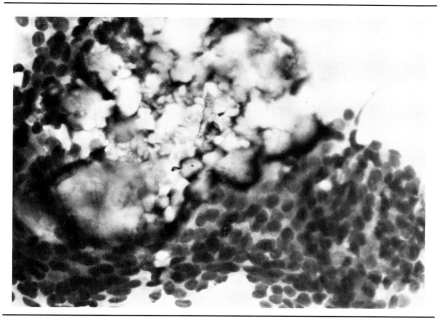

Figure 11.46.
Carcinoma with multinucleated giant cells. A group of epithelial cells with a large calcific deposit in the center (×400).

Squamous Cell Carcinoma

We have seen one case of this rare tumor. The patient was a 48-year-old black woman who was referred to a surgeon with a "recently discovered" 7-cm right breast mass. He aspirated 6 ml of orange-brown fluid. Smears from reaspiration of the residual mass revealed abundant proteinaceous material in the background with many hemosiderin-laden macrophages, polymorphonuclear leukocytes, and needle-shaped cholesterol crystals. Clumps and irregular groups of malignant epithelial cells were present, some of which were very large and thick with occasional variation in nuclear size and shape (Fig. 11.47), and there were some loose atypical cells. Although it was not difficult at all to diagnose the malignancy, there was a relative paucity of cells in the smears. Some of the epithelial cells showed delicate and pale cytoplasm (Figs. 11.48 and 11.49) while others had dense and blue cytoplasm. Some cells tended to form whorls or "pearls" (Fig. 11.49). Atypical squamous cells with pyknotic nuclei were identified (Fig. 11.50). Characteristic clumps of dark blue necrotic material with a cloudy or glassy appearance were observed, quite different from the necrosis seen in comedocarcinoma. Ghosts of squamous cells were identified in the necrotic debris (Fig. 11.50).

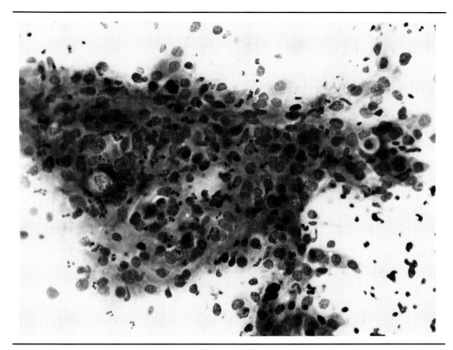

Figure 11.47.
Squamous cell carcinoma. Large thick cluster of neoplastic cells (×200).

Figure 11.48.
Squamous cell carcinoma. Clusters of loosely cohesive cells with delicate cytoplasm (×200).

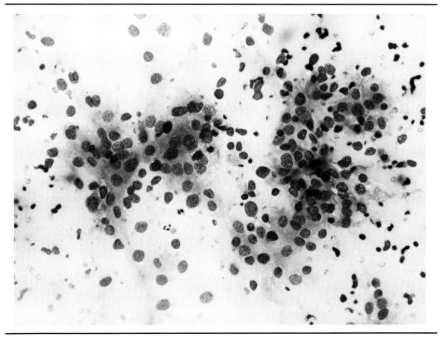

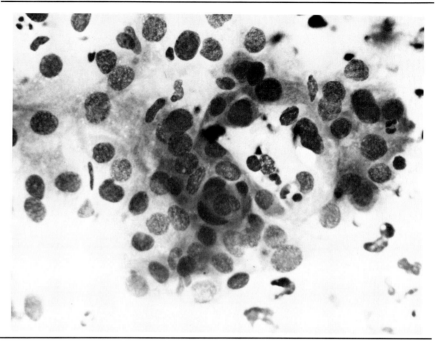

Figure 11.49.
Squamous cell carcinoma. Notice the cells arranged in a whorl (×400).

Figure 11.50.
Squamous cell carcinoma. Neoplastic cells with pyknotic nuclei and keratinized cyto-
plasm. Necrotic debris and ghosts of squamous cells are seen in the background (×400).

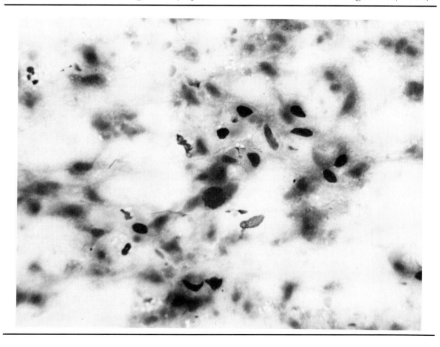

Paget's Disease

The smears obtained from patients with Paget's disease are not particularly cellular. They show abundant proteinaceous and necrotic debris in the background and some cholesterol crystals (Fig. 11.51). Many foamy histiocytes are observed, some with hemosiderin granules in the cytoplasm (Figs. 11.51 and 11.52). Occasional polymorphonuclear leukocytes are seen. Scattered throughout the smears one observes predominantly atypical single cells, mononucleated or binucleated (Fig. 11.53). Their cytoplasm varies from dense to delicate and may have vacuoles. These large cells have a high nuclear/cytoplasmic ratio. The nuclei are mostly round and have prominent nucleoli. Some of the atypical cells form cohesive clusters of a relatively small size (Fig. 11.53). An occasional larger group of atypical epithelial cells (Fig. 11.54) can be seen.

Figure 11.51.
Paget's disease. The smears show a "dirty background," foamy histiocytes, and cholesterol crystals (×200).

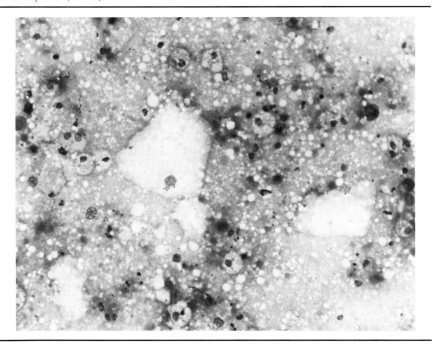

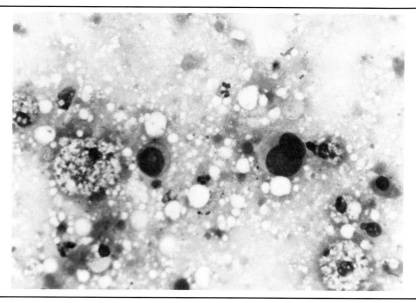

Figure 11.52.
Paget's disease. This photograph shows two markedly atypical epithelial cells (one is binucleated), some polymorphonuclear leukocytes, and hemosiderin-laden macrophages (×400).

Figure 11.53.
Paget's disease. This composite shows single atypical cells (top), *with high nuclear/ cytoplasmic ratio and small groups of cells with clearing of the cytoplasm* (bottom) *(×400).*

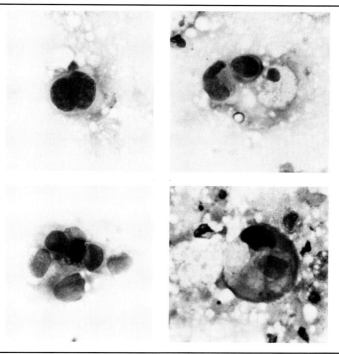

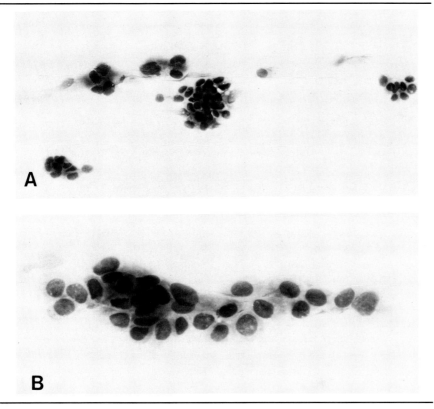

Figure 11.54.
Paget's disease. A. A few of the cellular clusters seen in this entity (×200). B. Higher magnification of one of the larger clusters (×400).

LOBULAR CARCINOMA

Lobular carcinomas are very fibrous and frequently gritty on aspiration. They can become quite large; hence multiple needles are inserted. However, at low magnification, the smears show very scant cellularity, and if one does not look at them closely, they may seem to show only blood. Under higher magnification some small groups of cells and single cells are observed (Figs. 11.55 and 11.56). The cells are somewhat larger than monocytes and their nuclei are round to slightly ovoid (Fig. 11.57). One may or may not see nucleoli. Sometimes the cytoplasm may show a large vacuole that displaces the nucleus toward one side (Fig. 11.57). The small cellular groups frequently are attached to fibrocollagenous tissue fragments and may show distorted nuclei. Again, we want to emphasize that under low power these cells are relatively inconspicuous. Be sure to screen the smears under higher magnification before reporting a case as unsatisfactory. This is a source of false negative diagnosis, particularly to inexperienced eyes.

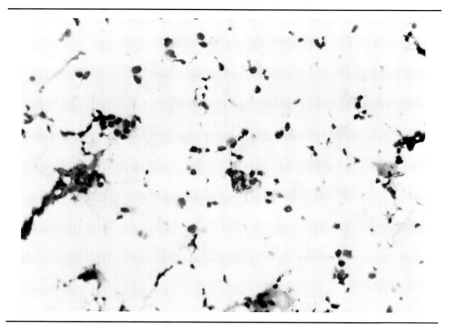

Figure 11.55.
Lobular carcinoma. Epithelial cells are scattered throughout the field, singly and in loosely cohesive small groups (×200). Although this is one of the most cellular areas we could find for photographic purposes, we still do not see the so-called tumor cellularity. This same field at (×100) magnification would show practically nothing. Also compare to Figures 10.1, 10.3, and 10.5 of ductal adenocarcinoma.

Figure 11.56.
Lobular carcinoma. Epithelial cells with small nuclei are scattered throughout. A small group with slightly enlarged nuclei shows a tendency to form an "Indian file." Notice that most of the cells in close relationship to the connective tissue show marked nuclear distortion and crush artifact (×200).

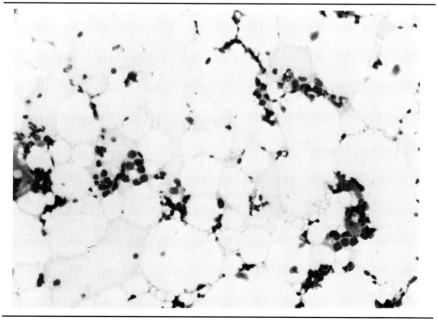

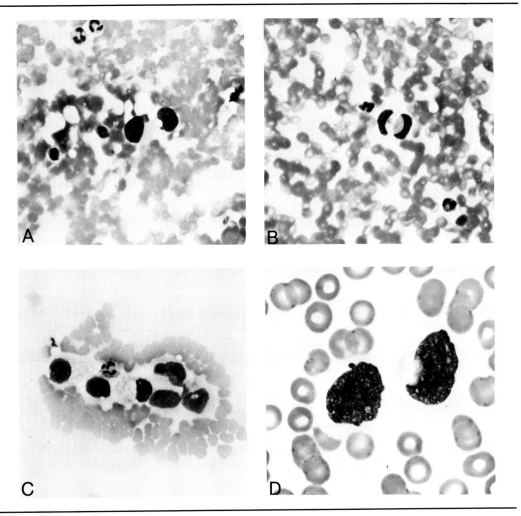

Figure 11.57.
Lobular carcinoma. This composite shows the occasional slightly enlarged epithelial cell that can be easily overlooked. Notice the hemorrhagic background and compare the size of the cells to that of the erythrocytes or lymphocytes (A, B, C ×400; D ×1,000). In the upper right panel two cells with nuclei molded around a vacuole are seen (×400). Two atypical cells with very scant cytoplasm are seen in the lower right panel (×1000).

We have observed three additional cytologic patterns in lobular carcinoma:

1. Sheets and/or clumps of ductal epithelial cells resembling those observed in ductal hyperplasia (Fig. 11.58)—the only difference is that these are seen in postmenopausal women.
2. Many "balls" of slightly enlarged epithelial cells with some loss of cohesiveness (Fig. 11.59)—some of these nuclei display nucleoli.
3. A few markedly atypical epithelial cells (Fig. 11.60)—due to the lack of tumor cellularity, in such cases we do not make a definite diagnosis of carcinoma.

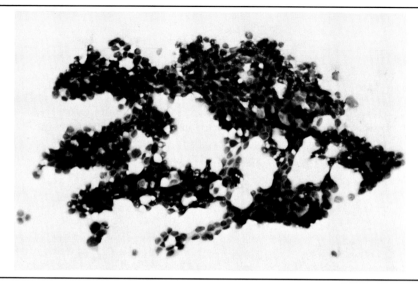

Figure 11.58.
Lobular carcinoma. Irregular thick clump of epithelial cells with fingerlike projections reminiscent of ductal hyperplasia (×200).

Figure 11.59.
Lobular carcinoma. This composite shows the atypical epithelial cells arranged in loosely cohesive "balls" or groups. Compare the size of the neoplastic nuclei to the size of the erythrocytes (A and B ×400). Sometimes the groups of cells are elongated (C ×400); some may show cytoplasmic vacuoles (D ×1000). Please compare with Figure 6.5.

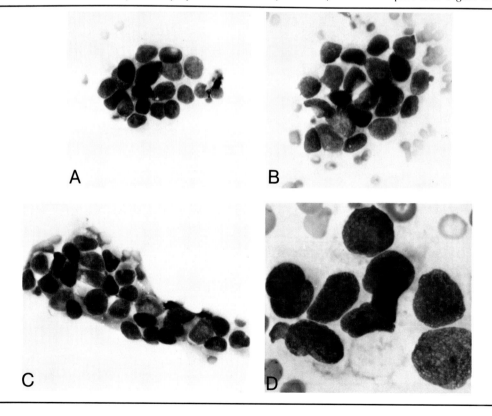

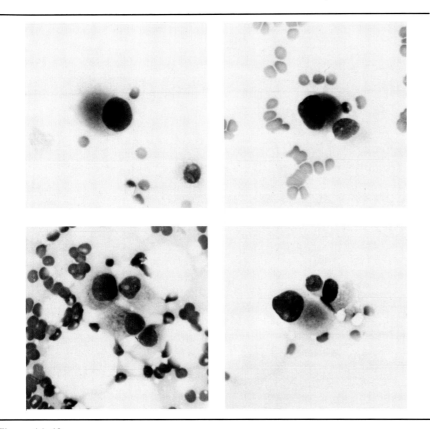

Figure 11.60.
Lobular carcinoma. This composite shows the enlarged atypical cells (singly and in small groups) suggestive of ductal adenocarcinoma (×400). Compare with Figure 11.57.

Our experience suggests that infiltrating lobular carcinoma will very seldom show tumor cellularity. In a few instances we have observed very cellular smears and the histology has revealed both infiltrating and in situ lobular carcinoma. The in situ component has been the predominant element.

CARCINOMA IN UNUSUAL HOSTS

Ductal Carcinoma in Pregnancy

Cytologically these are virtually indistinguishable from those seen in the non-pregnant patient except for some clusters of benign epithelial cells with lactational changes.

Ductal Carcinoma of the Male Breast

Cytologically they are exactly the same as cases of ductal carcinoma in the female.

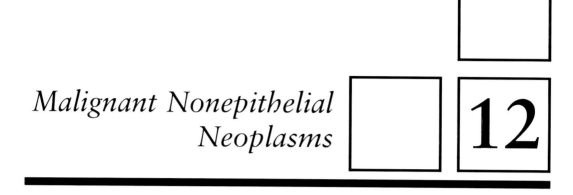

Malignant Nonepithelial Neoplasms

12

LEUKEMIA AND LYMPHOMA

These lesions bleed very easily and the patients immediately develop hematomas. Sometimes there is a history of leukemia or lymphoma; at other times the primary diagnosis will be determined after the fine needle aspiration. In both instances, the smears are extremely cellular, and there is marked cellular fragility. In leukemia, under higher magnification, marked variations in the cellular population are evident (Fig. 12.1). Some have irregular nuclei, others have round nuclei; some have cytoplasmic granules. In cases of lymphoma, there is a more monotonous infiltrate (Fig. 12.2). Sometimes the nuclei have protrusions. In both entities there are occasional clusters of benign ductal cells scattered throughout the smears (Fig. 12.3).

MYCOSIS FUNGOIDES

An elderly woman with mycosis fungoides developed a firm breast mass that was suspected to be breast cancer. The aspirates were cellular and reminiscent of malignant lymphoma; the cells, most of which were single ones, exhibited fragility. The occasional cellular clusters had the appearance of "lymphoid tangles" (Fig. 12.4). In some of the better-preserved groups, which were relatively small, there was marked variation in nuclear size and shape. Most of these cells were easily identifiable as nonepithelial (Fig. 12.5). Some polymor-

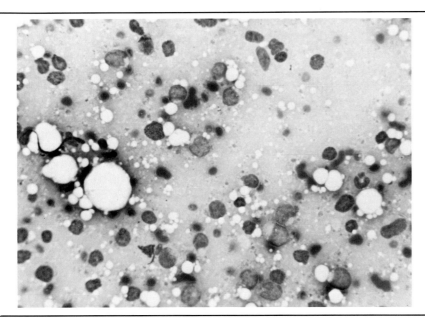

Figure 12.1.
Leukemia. Myeloid cells in different stages of maturation seen in a proteinaceous background (×400).

Figure 12.2.
Lymphoma. Large numbers of lymphoid cells with variable nuclear sizes (small and large lymphocytes) and different intensities of nuclear staining. Notice the delicate cytoplasm of some of the cells and the crush artifact (nuclear strands) (×400).

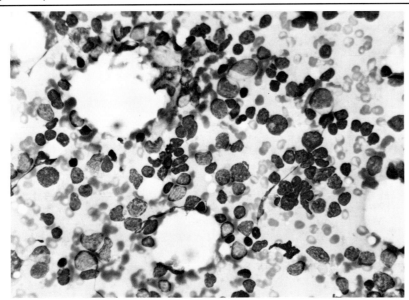

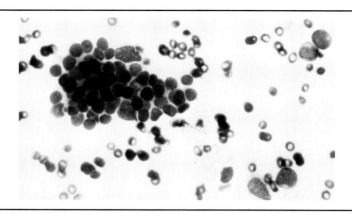

Figure 12.3.
Leukemia. Cluster of benign ductal cells with small regular nuclei and adjacent immature myeloid cells (×400).

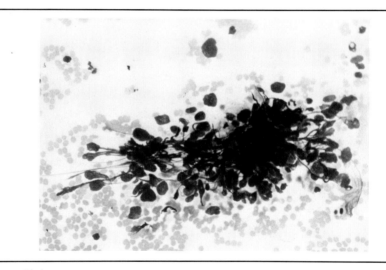

Figure 12.4.
Mycosis fungoides. "Lymphoid tangle" due to marked nuclear fragility (×200).

phonuclear leukocytes and lymphocytes of different sizes were seen. Some lymphoid cells adopted very bizarre shapes (Fig. 12.6). In general, their cytoplasm was either not evident or very delicate. A few nucleoli were observed.

The patient responded to radiation treatment and the mass disappeared. Needless to say, no excisional biopsy was necessary.

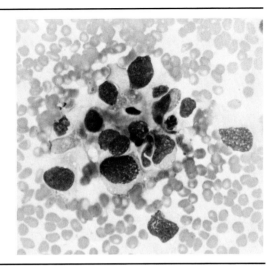

Figure 12.5.
Mycosis fungoides. A small, well-preserved, non-epithelial cell group. Notice the variation in nuclear size and the spireme appearance of some of the nuclei (×400).

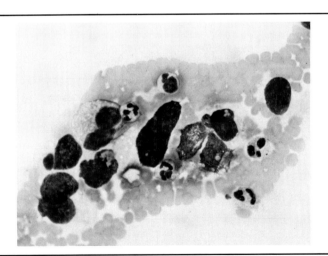

Figure 12.6.
Mycosis fungoides. Lymphoid cells with marked variation in nuclear size and shape. Most of them are devoid of cytoplasm (×400).

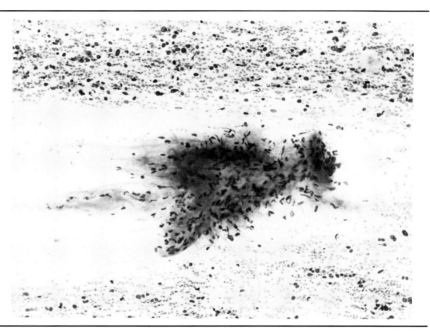

Figure 12.7.
Cystosarcoma phyllodes. Large, very cellular fibrocollagenous tissue fragment and naked nuclei of variable sizes in the background (×100).

Figure 12.8.
Cystosarcoma phyllodes. Extremely cellular, loose, fibrocollagenous tissue fragment (×100).

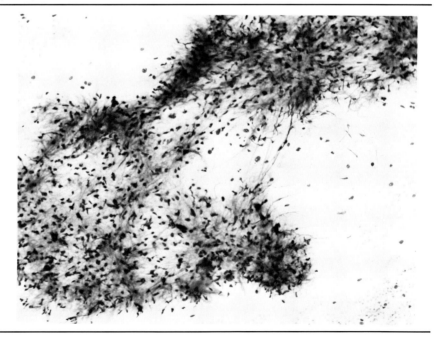

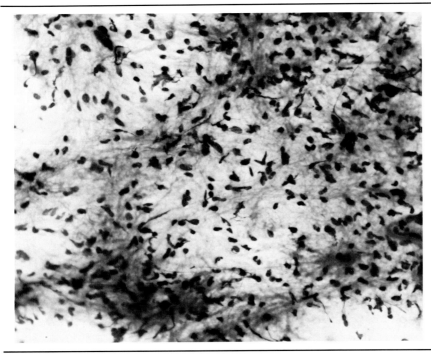

Figure 12.9.
Cystosarcoma phyllodes. Higher magnification of the fibrocollagenous tissue reveals the loose edematous, fibrillary arrangement and the variation in nuclear size and shape (×200).

CYSTOSARCOMA PHYLLODES

The lesions vary in size from relatively small to 15 cm or more in diameter. The smears are reminiscent of those seen in fibroadenoma. The sheets of epithelial cells are quite similar. In both instances there are many stripped bipolar nuclei in the background. In cases of cystosarcoma, these nuclei tend to vary in size and shape (Fig. 12.7), and some may adopt bizarre shapes. The differential diagnosis rests on the presence of fibrous connective tissue. In cases of cystosarcoma, this fibrous connective tissue is very loose and has large numbers of fibroblasts with elongated nuclei (Figs. 12.7–12.9). Many blood vessels are seen in this connective tissue (see Color Plates XXIX and XXX).

Metastatic Tumors in the Breast

13

The incidence of metastatic tumors in the breast from other primary sites is rare (Nielsen et al. 1981); however, to avoid potential pitfalls, one should be aware of their occurrence.

MALIGNANT MELANOMA

In our experience the most frequent metastases have been from malignant melanoma. As a rule, these lesions bleed easily on aspiration. In contrast to the fresh, bright red blood obtained in leukemias and lymphomas and in some mammary carcinomas, the aspiration in cases of metastatic melanoma yields dark brown, thick blood. The smears are extremely cellular and usually two types of cells are observed: round cells with a moderate amount of cytoplasm and spindled cells, both of which display prominent nucleoli. Occasionally the metastasis will consist almost entirely of the round cells (Fig. 13.1). In most of our cases melanin has not been a conspicuous element. Most of the cells appear isolated or loosely cohesive and very seldom large, tight cell clusters may be seen. Mitoses are common, much more common than in any primary breast carcinoma (Figs. 13.1–13.3). The same applies to the presence of "intranuclear inclusions" (Figs. 13.2 and 13.3).

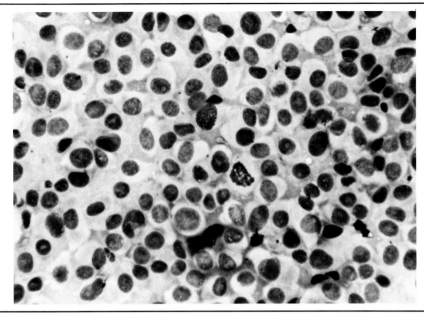

Figure 13.1.
Metastatic melanoma. Sheet of loosely cohesive neoplastic cells showing moderate variation in nuclear size. Note mitotic figure in the center of the field (×400).

Figure 13.2.
Metastatic melanoma. Two neoplastic cells showing prophase chromosomes. Also notice small intranuclear inclusion in upper left corner (×1000).

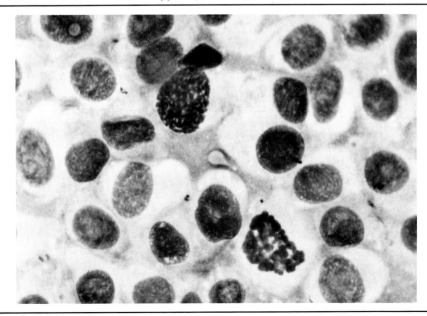

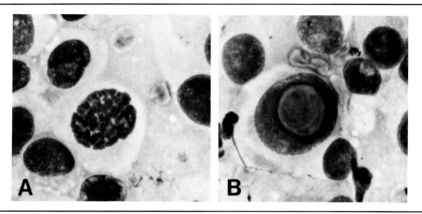

Figure 13.3.
Metastatic melanoma. A. Neoplastic cell with clear cytoplasm and prophase chromosomes (×1000). B. Neoplastic cell showing intranuclear inclusion. Mitoses and intranuclear inclusions are frequent findings in metastatic melanoma, much more frequent than in primary carcinomas of the breast (×1000).

RENAL CELL CARCINOMA

We have also seen a metastatic renal cell carcinoma in the breast. This lesion was aspirated by a surgeon, and we do not know how it felt on aspiration, but the smears were grossly hemorrhagic. After Diff-Quik staining, our first impression was that this had to be a neoplasm but it did not resemble any of the usual mammary carcinomas. We called the surgeon and requested the patient's clinical history after explaining that we knew we were dealing with a cancer but that we did not recognize the type. The surgeon mentioned that the patient had had a carcinoma of the uterine cervix two or three years previously and a renal cell carcinoma ten years ago. Immediately the clusters of pale foamy cells (Fig. 13.4–13.6) with prominent nucleoli made sense. Since this case we have seen several other renal cell carcinomas metastatic to the subcutis. They share the same cytologic features, often a "pink core" in the epithelial clusters (Color Plate XXXI) with most of the cells in large groups. Some cells lie singly, and occasionally some are spindled.

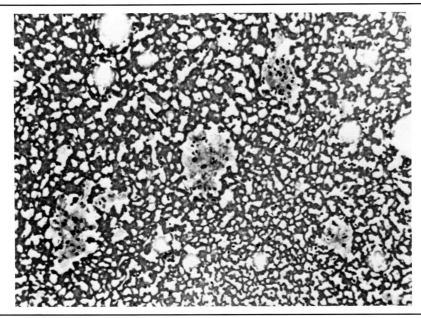

Figure 13.4.
Metastatic renal cell carcinoma. A few clusters of cells scattered in a hemorrhagic background (×100).

Figure 13.5.
Metastatic renal cell carcinoma. A cluster of epithelial cells with delicate cytoplasm, some cells with very small vacuoles, and nuclei with slight variation in size and shape. Notice some well-defined cell borders (×400).

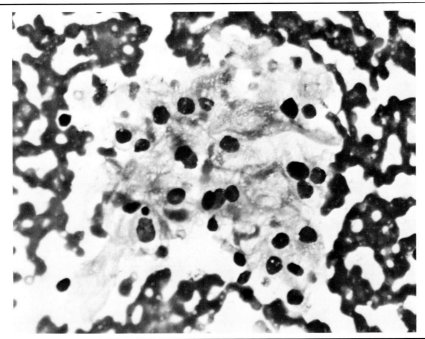

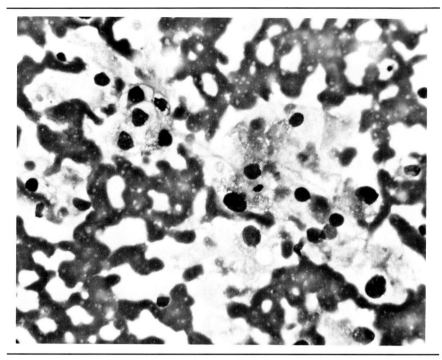

Figure 13.6.
Metastatic renal cell carcinoma. Another group of epithelial cells with ample, delicate, finely vacuolated cytoplasm. These cells show more variation in the nuclear size. Notice the hemorrhagic background (×400).

Carcinomas of the thyroid, colon, lung, esophagus, stomach, and an ileal carcinoid have been reported also, as the primary neoplasms metastasizing to the breast (Nielsen et al. 1981). Usually when the breast mass is discovered, the patient has widespread metastases and the diagnosis is not difficult. However, in some instances, the breast mass is the first indication of an "occult primary." Recognition of the lesion as metastatic will avoid an unnecessary mastectomy.

Thoracic Wall Recurrences and Axillary Masses

14

Recurrent or metastatic mammary carcinoma in the chest wall is easy to diagnose on fine needle aspiration except in cases of lobular carcinoma. Clinically, they can present as single or multiple subcutaneous nodules, sometimes along the scar from the previous mastectomy. When the smears are scanty, it might be necessary to change to a 23- or a 25-gauge needle. Fragments of fibroadipose tissue frequently are seen, and in close proximity to them are numerous atypical epithelial cells that lie in clusters or singly (Figs. 14.1 and 14.2). At higher magnification, the nuclear pleomorphism is evident (Fig. 14.2B).

AXILLARY LYMPH NODE METASTASES

It is a standard procedure in our service to examine the axillae of any patient who comes with a mass in the breast. If an axillary mass is discovered, we aspirate it after requesting the patient's permission and explaining that her cooperation is most essential. If the patient moves, aspirating the node will be difficult, much more difficult than if one were aspirating a tumor in the breast. These axillary aspirates are done more easily if the patient is sitting up and has the ipsilateral hand on her hip or on the shoulder of the cytotechnologist. A word of caution: axillary aspirations can cause pneumothorax. Aspirate while the patient is exhaling and then ask her not to breathe so that you can go deeper into the nodule without any fear of entering the chest cavity and tearing pleura and pulmonary parenchyma.

Lymph nodes with metastatic carcinoma are the easiest smears to diagnose.

161

At low magnification, there are many markedly atypical epithelial cells, arranged singly and in clusters, mixed with the small lymphoid cells.

Occasionally we have had cases in which there were no palpable mammary masses, but aspiration of an axillary nodule yielded a metastatic breast carcinoma.

We also have had cases that clinically mimicked carcinoma of the breast with axillary lymph node metastasis and then were discovered to be benign. Such a case is one we have already mentioned, in which an erosive lesion of the nipple was thought to be Paget's disease but the smears showed herpesvirus infection (Figs. 8.26–8.29). The axillary mass did not contain any metastasis; instead, reactive lymphadenitis secondary to the viral process was present. In another instance in which a patient had both a mammary and an ipsilateral axillary mass, the aspiration revealed fat necrosis of the breast and, in the axillary nodule, large numbers of foamy histiocytes (Figs. 14.3 and 14.4), and occasional lipogranulomas. The lesions disappeared after two weeks of symptomatic treatment with hot pads. In retrospective questioning of this patient, she admitted jumping rope without wearing a brassiere. She had large breasts and two days after jumping rope she noticed the tender lesion in the breast. The surgeon who saw her discovered the axillary mass and aspirated both masses.

Figure 14.1.
Recurrent mammary carcinoma in the thoracic wall. A group of adipose tissue cells is surrounded by atypical epithelial cells (×200).

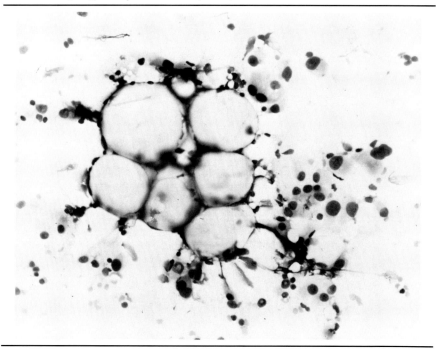

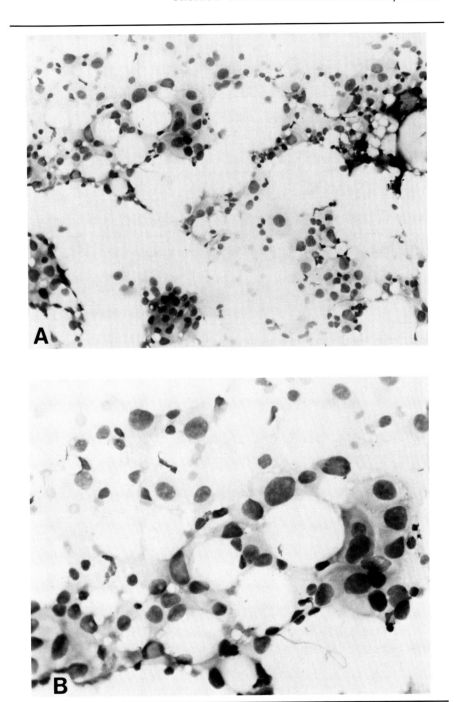

Figure 14.2.
Metastatic mammary carcinoma in the chest wall. Notice tumor cellularity and marked variation in nuclear size. Some of these cells are infiltrating fibroadipose tissue (A, upper right corner), *others tend to form glandular lumina. A. (×200). B. (×400).*

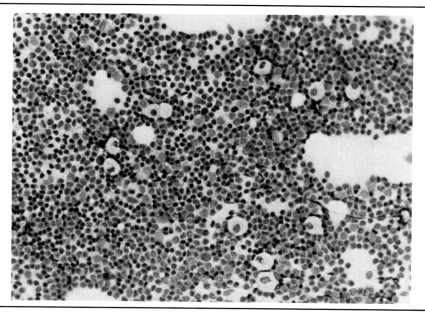

Figure 14.3.
Hyperplastic axillary lymph node. This patient had fat necrosis of the breast. The axillary lymph node showed large numbers of foamy histiocytes and occasional lipogranulomas (×200).

Figure 14.4.
Hyperplastic axillary lymph node. This is a higher magnification than Figure 14.3 to show the cellular detail. Notice the small and large lymphocytes, the foamy histiocytes, and the occasional plasma cells (×400).

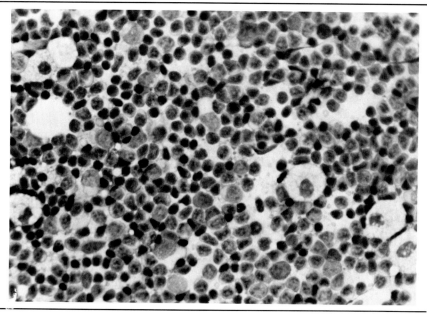

NEOPLASMS OF NERVOUS TISSUE

Schwannomas or neurilemomas can present as axillary masses and clinically be mistaken for a lymph node metastasis. On aspiration this is one of the few

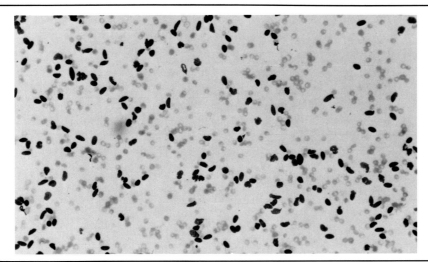

Figure 14.5.
Schwannoma or neurilemoma. Very cellular smears consisting predominantly of stripped, ovoid to cigar-shaped nuclei (×200).

Figure 14.6.
Schwannoma or neurilemoma. Large tissue fragments of variable thickness. At the lower left there are so many superimposed cells that cellular detail is not evident (×100).

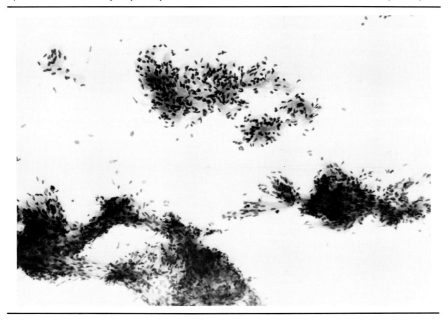

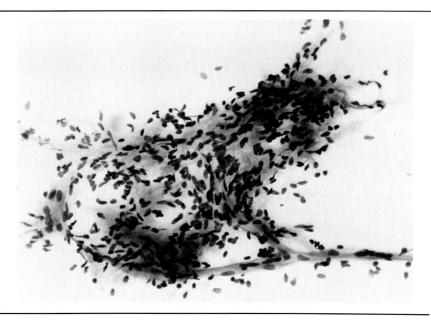

Figure 14.7.
Schwannoma or neurilemoma. This irregular fragment shows a moderate amount of connective tissue and many ovoid nuclei. Notice the branching capillary on the lower right (×200).

instances in which the procedure will be very painful. The patient will complain immediately of sharp pain that radiates to her fingers. The smears are quite cellular and exhibit many stripped ovoid nuclei (Fig. 14.5) and clumps of cells in a parallel or "palisading" arrangement (Fig. 14.6; Color Plate XXXII). There are also loose disorganized fragments of pink-staining connective tissue, sometimes traversed by capillaries (Fig. 14.7).

ACCESSORY MAMMARY TISSUE IN AXILLA

See Chapter 8 for a discussion of this entity.

Pitfalls ☐ **15**

ORGANIZING HEMATOMA

If the trauma causing the hematoma occurred in the remote past, the patient will not remember it. Clinically the lesion may resemble carcinoma. On aspiration, dark brown, thick material is obtained. The smears show lysed red blood cells, cholesterol crystals, amorphous debris, multinucleated giant cells, histiocytes (some with foamy cytoplasm, others with hemosiderin pigment), and some atypical cells. The degree of atypia of the single cells can be marked. The nucleus may be very large and irregular. Sometimes the nucleolus is conspicuous (Fig. 15.1). In one of our cases these atypical cells had bluish to black pigment in the cytoplasm. We misinterpreted this as a metastatic malignant melanoma (Oertel and Galblum 1983, pp. 400–401). To complicate matters, some of the cells are round while others are spindled, as one would expect in a metastatic melanoma. However, there is no tumor cellularity (Color Plate IV).

HERPETIC INFECTION OF THE NIPPLE

This case clinically resembled Paget's disease of the nipple. In addition it was accompanied by an axillary mass thought to represent a lymph node metastasis. The smears showed bizarre cells that can be misdiagnosed as malignant cells (Fig. 8.27).

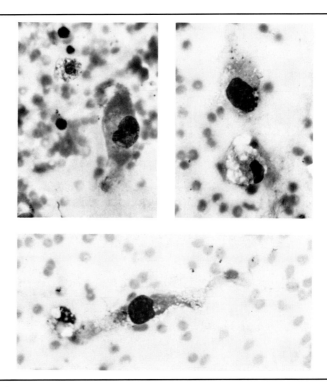

Figure 15.1.
Organizing hematoma. This is a composite of the atypical cells found in our only false positive case in this series. These cells have variable shapes, some cytoplasmic granules, prominent nucleoli, and enlarged nuclei (this is quite evident when compared to the size of the erythrocytes) (×400).

GRANULAR CELL TUMOR VERSUS DUCTAL ECTASIA

We made a mistake that easily could have been avoided if the pathologist had seen and aspirated the patient. Submitted smears showed large numbers of cells with foamy and/or granular cytoplasm (Figs. 15.2 and 15.3) with small nuclei and prominent nucleoli. They covered almost the entire slide. We interpreted this as "tumor cellularity, most consistent with granular cell myoblastoma." The lesion was excised and revealed marked ductal ectasia. The vacuolated and "granular" cells were histiocytes. All the cases of granular cell myoblastoma that we have seen subsequently (both in the breast and in the soft tissue) do not have well-preserved cell membranes. These cells are very fragile and if extreme care is not exercised when making the smears, all that is evident are naked nuclei with prominent nucleoli and a dirty granular background (Color Plates XIV and XV). The presence of multinucleated histiocytes is most consistent with ductal ectasia (Fig. 8.9); we have not seen multinucleated histiocytes in granular cell myoblastoma.

PAS (periodic acid–Schiff) stain, with and without diastase digestion, will not help in the differential diagnosis. Both the histiocytes and the granular cells will stain positively with PAS technique and will be resistant to diastase digestion.

Fig
Fa
an
ad

Figure 15.2.
Ductal ectasia. Very cellular smears with large numbers of loosely cohesive clear cells. This can be misinterpreted as tumor cellularity (×100).

Figure 15.3.
Ductal ectasia. Sheet of foamy histiocytes with slight variation in nuclear size (×400). Compare this to the illustrations of granular cell myoblastoma (Figs. 8.42 and 8.43).

Sm
no
an

Th
19
ko
cel
nu
str
an
(Fi

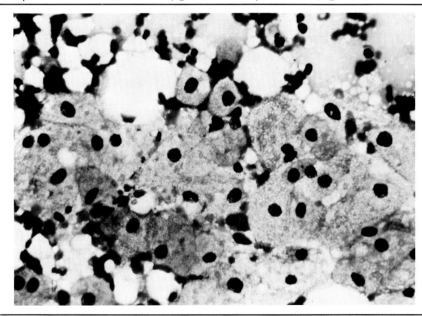

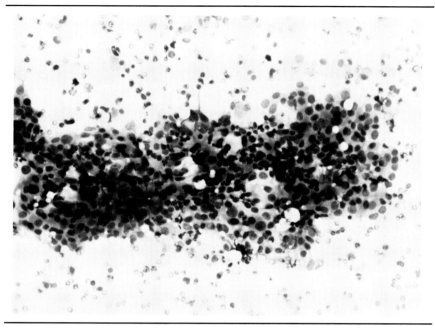

Figure 15.6.
Abscess with atypical cells. Large group of ductal epithelial cells that even at this low magnification show moderate variation in nuclear size and a tendency to form glandular lumina (×200).

Figure 15.7.
Abscess with atypical cells. Large irregular group of moderately atypical epithelial cells and some loose cells (upper right corner), *with prominent nucleoli (×200).*

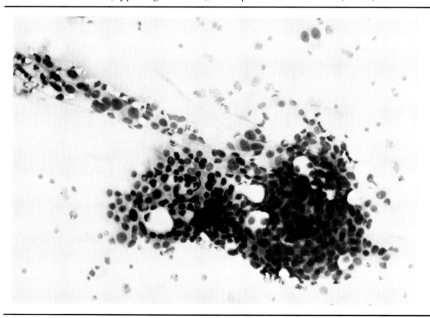

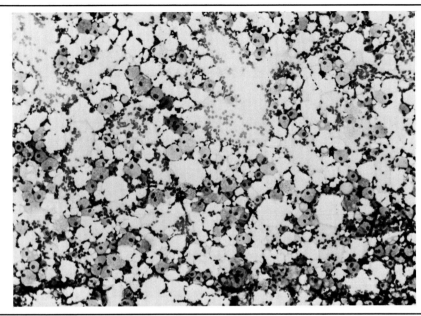

Figure 15.2.
Ductal ectasia. Very cellular smears with large numbers of loosely cohesive clear cells. This can be misinterpreted as tumor cellularity (×100).

Figure 15.3.
Ductal ectasia. Sheet of foamy histiocytes with slight variation in nuclear size (×400). Compare this to the illustrations of granular cell myoblastoma (Figs. 8.42 and 8.43).

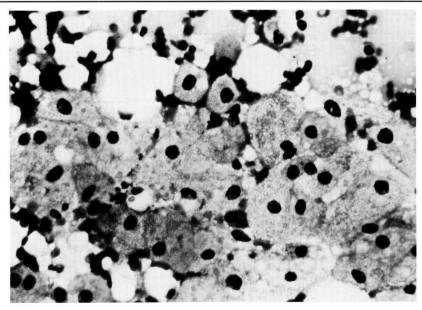

FAT NECROSIS

Clinically fat necrosis can mimic carcinoma. On aspiration the smears are thick and show large numbers of different sized vacuoles, many histiocytes, and some inflammatory cells. The clumps of epithelial cells may exhibit some atypia (Figs. 15.4 and 15.5) and are a source of false positive diagnosis (Magarey and Watson 1976, p. 348). The lack of tumor cellularity should prevent this from happening. However, fat necrosis may coexist with breast carcinoma or be adjacent to it; therefore you might sample the fat necrosis and not reach the adjacent carcinoma. In this case, fat necrosis is a source of false negative diagnosis. Based on the old premise of "first do no harm," we approach these cases in a cautious, prudent manner. If the fat necrosis does not resolve in a reasonable period of time (two to three weeks), then the lesion must be excised surgically.

Figure 15.4.
Fat necrosis with atypical cells. Large irregular group of ductal epithelial cells adjacent to a focus of fat necrosis. Notice the marked cellularity of the smear (×200).

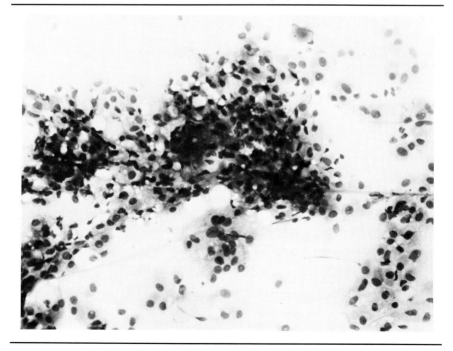

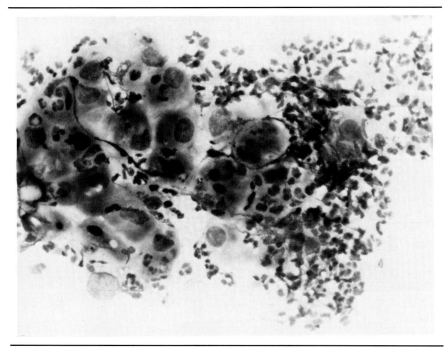

Figure 15.5.
Fat necrosis with atypical cells. Sheet of ductal epithelial cells with some apocrine changes and moderate variation in nuclear size. Notice large numbers of inflammatory cells adjacent to the epithelial cells (×400).

COMEDOMASTITIS

Smears reveal abundant necrotic debris indistinguishable from comedocarcinoma. The numerous clusters of cells that occur exhibit slight atypia (Figs. 8.10 and 8.11) that may be a source of false positive diagnosis.

ACUTE MASTITIS AND ABSCESS

These entities have been reported as a cause of false positive diagnosis (Frable 1976, pp. 172–173). The smears show innumerable polymorphonuclear leukocytes, and some lymphocytes and histiocytes. Variable numbers of epithelial cell clusters are observed (Color Plate VII), and sometimes they are quite numerous. They vary in size and thickness and some tend to form glandular structures (Figs. 15.6 and 15.7). Atypical single cells may be present (Fig. 15.7) and at higher magnification the nuclear pleomorphism is appreciated readily (Figs. 15.8 and 15.9).

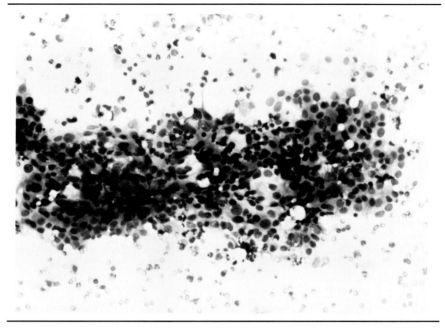

Figure 15.6.
Abscess with atypical cells. Large group of ductal epithelial cells that even at this low magnification show moderate variation in nuclear size and a tendency to form glandular lumina (×200).

Figure 15.7.
Abscess with atypical cells. Large irregular group of moderately atypical epithelial cells and some loose cells (upper right corner), *with prominent nucleoli (×200).*

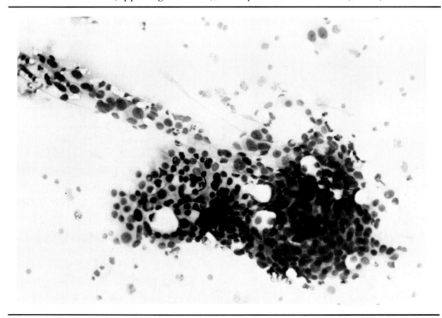

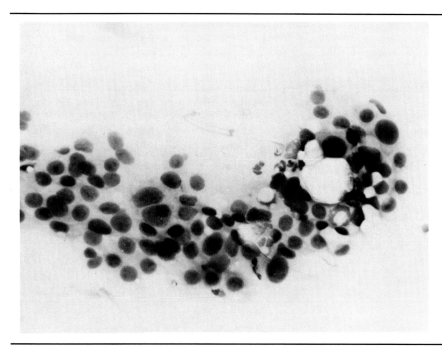

Figure 15.8.
Abscess with atypical cells. Thick cluster showing moderate variation in nuclear size and shape and some conspicuous nucleoli. Notice glandular lumen (×400).

Figure 15.9.
Abscess with atypical cells. Epithelial cells with marked variation in nuclear size. Notice that the cells are losing cohesiveness (×400).

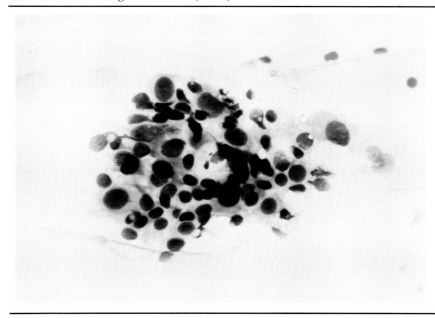

FIBROADENOMAS

Fibroadenomas are the most frequent cause of false positive diagnoses. As a rule these smears are very cellular. If there is little fibrous connective tissue and the aspirate has not been performed by the pathologist, the possibility of atypical ductal hyperplasia is entertained. To suggest this diagnosis the sheets and clusters of cells should not be particularly cohesive and there should be some variation in nuclear size. This will be further complicated by the presence of atypical single cells. Interpreting these findings as atypical ductal hyperplasia is not a serious problem but diagnosing a fibroadenoma as a carcinoma is a major mistake. Table 15.1 may help with the differential diagnosis. One should keep in mind that when a carcinoma is present, most of the cells are atypical. Very seldom will one encounter benign ductal cells alternating with malignant cells in

Table 15.1
Morphological criteria to help differentiate between fibroadenoma and adenocarcinoma

Criteria	Fibroadenoma	Ductal Adenocarcinoma
Tumor cellularity.	Present.	Present.
Sheets of cells.	Many, large and folded. Uniform cells with regular nuclei and scant cytoplasm arranged in a monolayer, honeycomb appearance. Myoepithelial cells easily seen. Hundreds of nuclei per sheet.	Some, varied sizes and shapes. Nonuniform cells, variable nuclear sizes and amount of cytoplasm, loosely cohesive, and irregularly arranged. No myoepithelial cells. Fewer but larger nuclei in similar surface area.
Clumps of cells.	Blunt branching.	Irregular clumps of variable thickness.
Nuclei.	Small and regular.	Variable size and shape, some bizarre.
Single epithelial cells.	Rare.	Many.
Apocrine cells.	Sometimes present.	Usually absent.
Naked nuclei.	Innumerable, ovoid, no nucleoli.	Many, varied size and shape, easily visualized nucleoli.
Fibrous tissue.	Very abundant, some large fragments.	Rarely seen, small fragments.
Background.	Proteinaceous or clear.	Hemorrhagic, necrotic, or inflammatory.
Cellular atypia.	Rare; some single cells, or only a few at the periphery of a cell cluster.	Marked; many single cells, or entire cellular clusters.

the same clump or cluster, or groups of benign ductal cells mixed with groups of neoplastic cells, although this can happen when the tumor is small and the needle has gone through it into normal adjacent parenchyma. Needless to say, if the pathologist performs the aspiration there will be fewer problems in the interpretation of such smears.

Fibroadenoma in Pregnant Patients

The patient may or may not have been aware of a preexisting mass that suddenly increased in size.

On aspiration the lesions bleed easily. The smears are markedly cellular and the sheets of epithelial cells are large and may show variation in nuclear size. Some loosely cohesive cells with moderately atypical nuclei are seen at the periphery of the cellular clusters. There are many fragments of loose, edematous connective tissue frequently traversed by branching capillaries (Figs. 15.10 and 15.11). This suggests cystosarcoma phyllodes; however, the loose connective tissue fragments show very few spindled nuclei, which is unlike the cystosarcoma phyllodes (Fig. 12.8).

Figure 15.10.
Fibroadenoma in a pregnant patient. The smears are very cellular and have a hemorrhagic background. The fibrocollagenous tissue fragments are very loose and edematous. The sheets of ductal cells may show some nuclear atypia (×100).

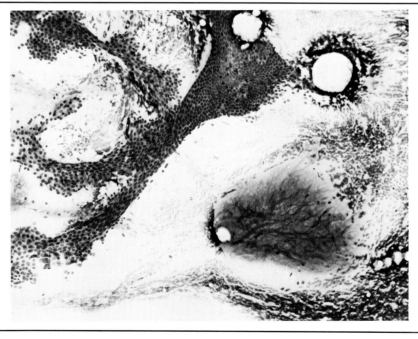

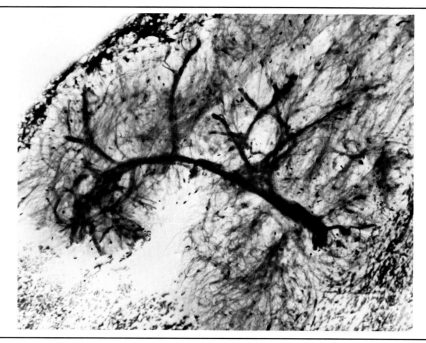

Figure 15.11.
Fibroadenoma in a pregnant patient. It is relatively common to find blood vessels in the loose, edematous fibrocollagenous tissue. This might raise the possibility of a cystosarcoma phyllodes, but as a rule the tissue fragments do not show many nuclei (×100).

Fibroadenoma in Elderly Women

As a rule, fibroadenomas are lesions of young women although we have seen some in women over 70 years of age. The smears can be very misleading—again the problem arises when one is dealing with submitted smears rather than smears obtained from an aspiration performed by oneself. Cellular smears always should be a cause of concern in elderly patients.

Atypical Fibroadenomas

Fibroadenomas become troublesome to diagnose when the stromal component is missing and the epithelial component is exuberant. The smears show tumor cellularity but the cords and sheets of cells are tightly cohesive (Fig. 15.12). Sometimes the nuclei are enlarged, although regular, and exhibit marked piling-up.

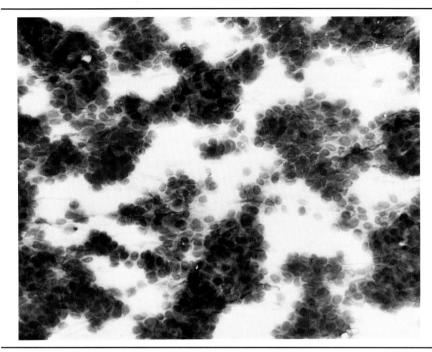

Figure 15.12.
*Atypical fibroadenoma. Numerous thick cords of epithelial cells with regular nuclei.
Notice absence of fibrocollagenous tissue (×200).*

In other cases the smears are very cellular, the epithelial cells show variation
in nuclear size; some are forming glandular structures and in addition single
enlarged cells are scattered throughout. These findings raise the possibility of
carcinoma (tumor cellularity, sheets of cells, and loose cells); however, the
marked cellular atypia of carcinoma in both the clusters and single cells is not
observed in fibroadenomas.

We have seen one case with bizarre multinucleated stromal giant cells that
had very delicate or no visible cytoplasm, and their nuclei were large and
irregular (usually two to four nuclei in each cell) (Figs. 15.13 and 15.14).
Nucleoli were prominent. Such stromal cells are strikingly different from the
multinucleated histiocytes one may occasionally see in fibroadenomas. Rosen
(1979a) called attention to their presence in benign conditions and pointed out
that they may be misinterpreted as invasive carcinoma of the breast.

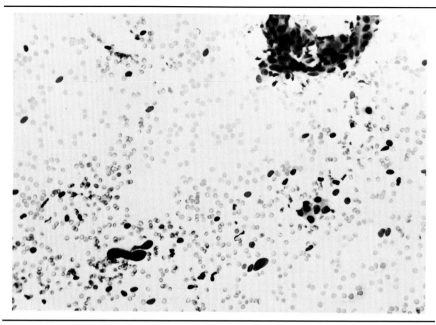

Figure 15.13.
Atypical fibroadenoma. One large cluster of epithelial cells, many stripped bipolar nuclei (darker and larger than the red blood cells in the background), and some bizarre nuclei (stromal giant cells) (×200).

Figure 15.14.
Atypical fibroadenoma. Notice the bizarre nuclei (from stromal giant cells), one adjacent to a fragment of collagenous tissue, the other close to a clump of ductal cells (×200).

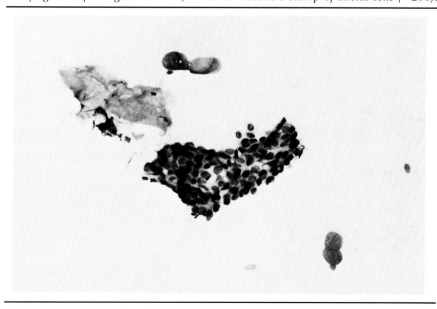

RADIATION-INDUCED ATYPIA

The problem consists of differentiating recurrent breast carcinoma from radiation-induced changes (see Table 15.2). Generally, there is a history of previous lumpectomy for carcinoma, axillary dissection, and radiation therapy. Underlying the surgical scar or adjacent to it is an ill-defined firmness. The smears show a proteinaceous background, fragments of fibroadipose tissue, and small numbers of generally single, markedly atypical cells. These bizarre cells (Fig. 15.15) have abundant delicate cytoplasm with vacuoles of varying size, and the nuclei are enlarged and irregular, some of which also display vacuoles. In some instances nucleoli can be observed. These are probably the atypical epithelial cells from the "terminal duct lobular unit" described by Schnitt et al. (1984, p. 545) or they may represent atypical fibroblasts. No tumor cellularity exists. Scattered throughout the smears are plump histiocytes with delicately vacuolated cytoplasm and enlarged nuclei (Fig. 15.16).

Table 15.2
Differential diagnosis between radiation-induced atypia and recurrent adenocarcinoma

	Radiation-induced Atypia	Recurrent Adenocarcinoma
On aspiration.	Rubbery.	Usually gritty.
After withdrawing the needle.	Easy bleeding, somewhat difficult to stop.	Some bleeding, easily stopped by applying pressure.
Smears.	Scant cellularity.	Tumor cellularity.
	Few single bizarre cells.	Many markedly atypical cells, singly and in clusters.
	Plump histiocytes.	Some foamy histiocytes.

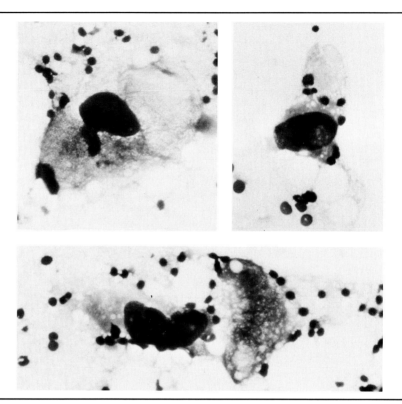

Figure 15.15.
Postradiation atypia. Single bizarre cells with large irregular nuclei and abundant, delicate, finely vacuolated cytoplasm (×400).

Figure 15.16.
Postradiation atypia. Foamy histiocytes (×400).

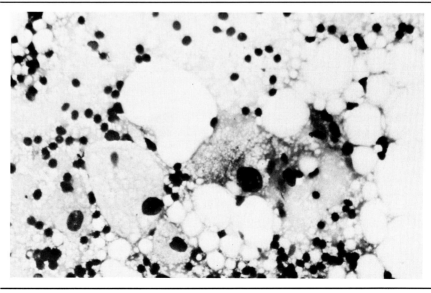

MISCONCEPTIONS

Probably the source of greatest apprehension for the surgeons is "seeding of the tumor in the needle tract." We believe that this is a myth. Even if it happened, that breast is going to be removed or will receive radiation therapy. This concern should have been put to rest long ago (McLean and Sugiura 1937; Söderström 1966, pp. 19–23; Zajicek 1974, pp. 191–192).

Fine Needle Aspiration of Nonpalpable Breast Lesions

16

We usually avoid performing aspirations on nonpalpable lesions evident only on mammograms and encourage the surgeons to perform excisional biopsies after radiologic localization. The 32 cases in which we have been persuaded to perform fine needle aspirations have made us reluctant to encourage this practice; only one carcinoma was detected. How have we approached them? First the physician or patient provides the mammograms ahead of the date of aspiration. These are shown to our radiologist, who then provides the coordinates needed for orientation. We are told how many centimeters to the right or left of the nipple, above or below the nipple (we will have an abscissa and an ordinate), and how deep we have to insert the needle to reach the lesion. Multiple aspirations of this region are performed, and as usual, one smear is checked after each aspirate. In summary, we believe it is a considerable effort, and we cannot be sure of precise localization.

In Sweden, ad hoc compression plates (Mühlow 1974) and stereotaxic needle aspirations (Bolmgren et al. 1977) of nonpalpable breast lesions have been performed for over ten years. These techniques are considered routine in some centers (Svane 1983; Svane and Silfverswärd 1983; Kehler and Albrechtsson 1984).

Feldman and Covell (1985, pp. 31–33) describe in detail and illustrate the procedure used at their institution, but they do not mention how many aspirates in their series belonged in the nonpalpable category or their rate of success. Kline et al. (1979, Table 4) reported seven cases of nonpalpable lesions aspirated by clinicians. In four of these, the aspirates were diagnosed as positive (for malignancy), one was suspicious, and two were negative. We are not told how the clinician localized the lesions.

Lately we have performed aspirates in four patients at the time the radiologist has placed the Kopans spring hook localizer needle. All of these samples have been unsatisfactory for cytologic diagnosis. This is a problem we need to solve.

The detection of nonpalpable breast malignancies is the greatest benefit of mammography. It is the trend of the future (Homer et al. 1984; Hall 1986), and I believe that their cytologic diagnosis poses the greatest challenge to fine needle aspiration.

Additional Diagnostic Information

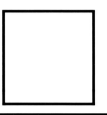

17

The consistency of a lesion and the gross appearance of an aspirate can yield useful clues.

CONSISTENCY OF LESION WHEN NEEDLING

1. Rubbery
   a. Fibrous mastopathy
   b. Fibroadenoma
2. Gritty (similar to inserting the needle in an apple)
   a. Ductal adenocarcinoma—Most aspirates will yield large numbers of cells. Excessive suction causes easy bleeding, particularly in scirrhous carcinoma, in which case the sample may consist predominantly of blood. Reaspirate less vigorously at the edge of the lesion (when you feel the change in consistency) to obtain tumor cellularity.
   b. Lobular adenocarcinoma—Generally the gritty consistency felt on aspiration is unmistakable, but the aspirate is scant, thin and watery, and no obvious diagnostic cells are seen when scanning the wet smear. No bleeding is observed, even when applying maximum suction (in contradistinction to ductal adenocarcinomas). Change to a smaller handle with a 10-cc syringe and a 23-gauge needle for a more generous sample.
3. Soft
   a. Lipoma and fatty replacement
   b. Medullary carcinoma
   c. Colloid carcinoma
   d. Adenoid cystic carcinoma

APPEARANCE OF SMEARS WITH THE NAKED EYE

1. Hemorrhagic smears
   a. Bright red blood
      Ductal adenocarcinoma
      Leukemia
      Metastatic renal cell carcinoma
   b. Dark brown blood
      Papillary adenocarcinoma of breast
      Metastatic melanoma
      Organizing hematoma
2. Thick mucoid smears
   a. Clear
      Colloid adenocarcinoma (subsequent aspirates will be mixed with blood
         as lesion bleeds easily)
      Adenoid cystic carcinoma
   b. Yellowish (pastelike)
      Abscess, suppurative mastitis
      Fat necrosis
      Subareolar abscess
      Comedomastitis
      Comedocarcinoma
3. Thin clear fluid
   a. Fibrocystic disease (variable amounts)
   b. Fibroadenoma (few drops)
   c. Lobular adenocarcinoma (few drops)

GUIDELINES FOR SMEAR EXAMINATION

1. Look for normal ductal cells and use them as a baseline, allowing for individual variation, because every aspirated breast will be slightly different.
2. Do not make a diagnosis on only one or two groups of cells or on an individual cell. Mistakes are made when interpreting cells in an isolated fashion, without considering the background in which they lie.
3. Nearly all neoplasias produce extremely cellular smears, the so-called tumor cellularity.
4. Rely on your experience as a surgical pathologist. For example, when examining histologic sections of elderly patients' breasts, you find "fatty replacement," fibrosis, and a very scant epithelial component. The same applies to aspiration smears.

GENERAL REMINDERS

1. We are extremely dependent on a *good sample*. If the lesion was missed, you will not make the right diagnosis. *Think before inserting the needle*, as

chances of success decrease with increasing numbers of needles, particularly with small lesions. Be patient and careful. Determine whether the lesion is more accessible to needling when the patient is sitting up or when the patient is lying down. If the latter position is less adequate, ask the patient to sit up again before performing the aspiration. The same applies for the position of the arms: determine whether it is better to have the patient's arm under the neck or at the side of the body. Remember that you, the operator, have to be in a comfortable position too. Accept responsibility for false negatives.

2. If surgeons or internists are performing the aspirations, make them aware of all the items discussed above. They will then have to assume responsibility for the false negatives.

3. When we make a diagnosis of carcinoma at our institution, the majority of surgeons will proceed with a mastectomy without a frozen section. This will probably become more prevalent throughout the country because of the emphasis on cost containment in the health-care field. Approach aspirations as you would a frozen section. When you are absolutely sure that there are malignant cells, say so. If you have the slightest doubt, request an excisional biopsy or a frozen section before proceeding with a mastectomy.

4. Despite all precautions, we are bound to make an occasional mistake. Try to keep in mind how your decisions affect a patient, and try to do no harm.

Statistical Summary

18

If a patient is referred to us with a mass in the breast, we also examine the axillae and the supraclavicular regions and aspirate any masses found. If the patient undergoes a mastectomy and a few years later develops a lesion of the chest wall that is aspirated, these aspirates have been included in this series as well.

We have entered 3,714 reports of aspirations (including 3 nipple discharges) performed or processed at The George Washington University Medical Center from 1976 through 1984 in an IBM-XT computer. Tables 18.1 through 18.10 show the data analyses we have obtained.

These 3,714 aspirates were performed on a total of 3,017 patients; 2,915 were women and 102 were men. The youngest patient was a 14-year-old girl and the oldest were two 94-year-old women. One "aspirate" equals one visit or one cytology report. Many of these reports represent sessions with the patients during which two to ten needles were inserted. A total of 393 patients have had two procedures at intervals ranging from a few days to several years. One patient has been followed for nine years with a total of fourteen visits for aspirations (Table 18.2).

The overall rate of unsatisfactory specimens was 17.3% (Table 18.3). When analyzing these figures by the specialty of the physician performing the fine needle aspiration, the pathologist has the best performance (Table 18.4). We would like to emphasize that "the pathologist" refers to pathology residents, fellows, and junior and senior staff.

Our findings confirm what had been reported long ago in the Swedish literature (Franzén and Zajicek 1968, p. 250), that optimal results are achieved when "the needling and the handling and the analysis of the smears are all done

Table 18.1
Analysis of fine needle aspirations based on location and diagnosis of lesion

Fine Needle Aspiration Site	Fine Needle Apiration Diagnosis				Total Aspirates
	Benign	Malignant	Inconclusive	Unsatisfactory	
Breast	2,104	618	243	640	3,605*
Axilla	23	42	4	2	71
Chest wall	6	29	0	0	35
Supraclavicular	0	3	0	0	3
Totals	2,133	692	247	642	3,714

*Includes three nipple discharges.

Table 18.2
Analysis of fine needle aspirations based on number of aspirates per patient

Number of Aspirates per Patient	Number of Patients	Cumulative Patients	Cumulative Aspirates
1	2,511	2,511	2,511
2	393	2,904	3,297
3	78	2,982	3,531
4	20	3,002	3,611
5	6	3,008	3,641
6	3	3,011	3,659
7	2	3,013	3,673
8	0	3,013	3,673
9	3	3,016	3,700
10	0	3,016	3,700
11	0	3,016	3,700
12	0	3,016	3,700
13	0	3,016	3,700
14	1	3,017	3,714
Totals		3,017	3,714

Table 18.3
Analysis of fine needle aspiration diagnosis according to the sex of the patient

Fine Needle Aspiration Diagnosis	Female	Male	Total Aspirates
Benign	2,056	77	2,133 (57.4%)
Malignant	682	10	692 (18.8%)
Inconclusive	245	2	247 (6.7%)
Unsatisfactory	624	18	642 (17.3%)

Table 18.4
Analysis of unsatisfactory aspirates according to physician's specialty

Physician's Specialty	Number of Aspirations Performed	Number of Unsatisfactory Aspirates	Percentage of Unsatisfactory Aspirates
Surgeon	2,238	510	22.8%
Pathologist	1,230	9	0.7%
Internist	246	123	50.0%

by the cytopathologist" (Zajicek 1974, p. 24). This has been also the experience of others (Zajdela et al. 1975, p. 500; Ingram et al. 1983, pp. 170−171).

The location of the lesions that were aspirated can be found in Table 18.5. In 75 aspirates it was not specified whether the lesion was on the right or left side. The great majority of these cases are from procedures performed in 1976 and 1977. Also, it is our policy that bilateral breast aspirates done on a patient during the same office visit are counted as one if the the aspirates have identical diagnoses (*e.g.*, fibrocystic disease). This generates only one bill, otherwise the patients would be charged for two aspirations.

In our series there were a few more carcinomas in the right breast than in the left (Table 18.6). However, the difference is not significant.

Table 18.5
Analysis of fine needle aspirations based on side of lesion

Fine Needle Aspiration Site	Right	Left	Not Specified	Bilateral	Total
Breast	1,685	1,742	74	104	3,605
Axilla	29	41	0	1	71
Chest wall	16	17	1	1	35
Supraclavicular	0	3	0	0	3
Totals	1,730	1,803	75	106	3,714

Table 18.6
Analysis of malignant fine needle aspirations based on side of lesion

Fine Needle Aspiration Site	Right	Left	Not Specified	Bilateral	Total
Breast	313	301	3	1	618
Axilla	18	24	0	0	42
Chest wall	11	16	1	1	29
Supraclavicular	0	3	0	0	3
Totals	342	344	4	2	692
Percentage	49.4%	49.7%	0.6%	0.3%	100%

Follow-up information has been obtained for virtually all malignant (Table 18.7) and inconclusive (Table 18.8) aspirates. However, as this book goes to press we have follow-up information available on 61% of benign aspirates and on 56% of unsatisfactory aspirates. The minimal clinical follow-up information has been 15 months.

FALSE NEGATIVES AND FALSE POSITIVES

Of the 2,133 benign aspirates, 452 had excisional biopsies (Table 18.9). A benign diagnosis was confirmed in 390 cases. Twelve cases were diagnosed as atypical hyperplasia.

In 50 instances the tissue diagnosis was malignant for an 8% false negative rate.

Of the 50 patients with false negative aspirates that underwent excisional biopsies (1) in 14 cases no frozen section was done; (2) in 11 cases the frozen

Table 18.7
Follow-up of 692 malignant aspirates

Number of Malignant Aspirates	Follow-up
618	Mastectomy, excisional biopsy, *etc.* (one false positive)
42	Radiation and/or chemotherapy
18	Expired of disease (no autopsy)
1	Expired of disease (autopsy done)
7	Refused treatment
6	Lost to follow-up

Table 18.8
Follow-up of 247 inconclusive aspirates

Number of Inconclusive Aspirates	Follow-up	
206	Biopsy	
	Benign	64
	Adenocarcinoma	118
	Atypical hyperplasia	20
	Lymphoma	2
	Cystosarcoma	2
33	Clinical follow-up (doctor's office visit, mammogram, *etc.*)	
3	Expired	
1	Refused treatment	
4	Lost to follow-up	

Table 18.9
Benign aspirates with available follow-up

Number of Benign Aspirates	Follow-up	
452	Biopsy	
	Benign	390
	Malignant	50
	Atypical hyperplasia	12
238	Reaspirated	
577	Clinical follow-up (doctor's office visit, mammogram, *etc.*)	
8	Expired (unrelated causes)	
2	Refused treatment	
36	Lost to follow-up	

Table 18.10
Unsatisfactory aspirates with available follow-up

Number of Unsatisfactory Aspirates	Follow-up	
131	Biopsy	
	Benign	90
	Malignant	37
	Atypical hyperplasia	4
124	Reaspirated	
97	Clinical follow-up (doctor's office visit, mammogram, *etc.*)	
1	Expired (pneumonia)	
6	Lost to follow-up	

section diagnosis was benign; (3) in 2 cases the frozen section diagnosis was deferred; (4) in 23 cases the frozen section was positive for cancer.

Of the fourteen cases in which no frozen section was done at the time of excisional biopsy, the permanent sections revealed

Three intraductal carcinomas
Two in situ lobular carcinomas
Two infiltrating lobular carcinomas
One tubular carcinoma
Six infiltrating ductal adenocarcinomas, of which one was microscopic and incidentally found

Of the eleven cases in which the frozen section was negative, the permanent sections revealed

Two infiltrating ductal carcinomas
One malignant cystosarcoma phyllodes
One tubular carcinoma
Two intraductal carcinomas
Five in situ lobular carcinomas

Of the two cases in which the frozen section diagnosis was deferred, the permanent sections showed infiltrating ductal adenocarcinoma.

Of the fifty false negative cases, only nine were performed by pathologists. Again we want to reiterate that residents, fellows, and junior and senior pathology staff are included in this category:

1. Two patients were senile and uncooperative. One of them could not be moved from the wheel chair to the examining table, so sampling was very difficult. In both instances excisional biopsies were recommended.
2. In two cases the false negative was the result of inexperience. In one instance the pathologist-in-training who performed the aspiration did not ask for help and missed the lesion. In the other case it was the inexperience of the pathologist reading the smears. The malignant cells were present on the slides but were misdiagnosed as benign.
3. One patient had very large breasts and the needle only reached a zone of fat necrosis. Considering the patient's age, an excisional biopsy was requested. The frozen section was also read as fat necrosis, but permanent sections revealed infiltrating ductal carcinoma.
4. One patient had a ductal carcinoma with multinucleated giant cells. The smears appear innocuous, particularly when one is not acquainted with the entity.
5. One patient had subareolar induration, extremely painful during aspiration, which limited the amount of material we could obtain.
6. One patient had a small fibroadenoma, and on excision an infiltrating ductal carcinoma was found adjacent to it.
7. One patient had synchronous carcinomas. After aspirating the right breast and diagnosing it as adenocarcinoma, the left breast was not as thoroughly sampled as it would have been had it been the only lesion.

We realize the inevitability of some false negative diagnoses since no test will be 100% accurate. However, we would like to reiterate our concern with the 8% false negative rate in our series and are acutely aware of the problems it may create. Any delay in treatment worsens the prognosis for the patient and can result in legal consequences for the physicians involved. We have discussed this thoroughly with the surgeons and internists who refer patients to us or who send us smears for interpretation.

1. If the aspirates are reported to be benign but the referring physician considers the lesion to be malignant on clinical examination, he may proceed to excisional biopsy or reaspiration, or, more frequently, he sends the patient to us for a reaspiration.

2. If the patient has a discrete solid mass, and the aspirates are reported to be benign without a more specific diagnosis (*e.g.*, lipoma, fibroadenoma, *etc.*) most frequently an excisional biopsy will be performed.
3. If the aspirates are benign and the patient is in the high-risk category for breast carcinoma or has an abnormal mammogram, an excisional biopsy is performed.
4. If the aspirates are benign and the patient is not at high risk for breast carcinoma, she will be followed clinically, radiologically and/or by repeated aspirations.
5. Generally, the physicians who practice within a short distance of the University Hospital ask the patients to bring their smears to our laboratory. If they suspect a carcinoma, they will call us to express this concern and to let us know that the patient has been warned that we might have to reaspirate the breast mass. While the patient waits, the smears are stained with Diff-Quik and read while still wet. If the diagnosis of malignancy is not obvious, we reaspirate the mass.
6. Since July 1985, the fellows or residents performing breast aspirations on patients 50 years old or older are not allowed to let the patient leave the aspiration room unless they have obtained material diagnostic of carcinoma. A staff pathologist (who will later sign the report) has to be consulted and assume the responsibility that the mass is probably benign. This has created minor problems, particularly with senior fellows, who feel that we do not trust their judgment. Time will tell whether we will continue to adhere to this policy or whether we will eventually discontinue it.

Of the 692 malignant aspirates we had one false positive diagnosis. A 35-year-old white man presented with a subareolar nodule in the left breast which was aspirated by a surgeon. The two smears we received showed a hemorrhagic background and some atypical cells (round and spindled). Some had cytoplasmic granules. We interpreted this as a "malignant lesion (most consistent with a metastatic melanoma), left breast." Three days later the lesion was excised under local anesthesia. Histologic sections revealed an organizing hematoma. On further questioning the patient denied any history of trauma. In retrospect we should not have made a diagnosis of malignancy as no tumor cellularity was evident. The cytoplasmic granules (misinterpreted as melanin) represented hemosiderin pigment (Table 18.7).

In 617 cases (Table 18.7) the cytologic diagnosis of malignancy was confirmed (excisional biopsy and subsequent mastectomy, mastectomy with or without frozen section, and lately lumpectomies). Two hundred twenty-six mastectomies have been performed without a frozen section. Forty-two patients received radiation and/or chemotherapy (cases of inflammatory carcinoma, leukemia, lymphoma, mycosis fungoides, breast cancer with distant metastases, chest wall recurrences, *etc.*). Nineteen patients died with metastatic disease, and an autopsy was performed in one but not in the other eighteen patients. Seven patients refused treatment. One patient, with a colloid carcinoma, has been on "nutritional therapy" for two years. Another patient who refused treatment died with metastatic disease. Six patients have been lost to follow-up.

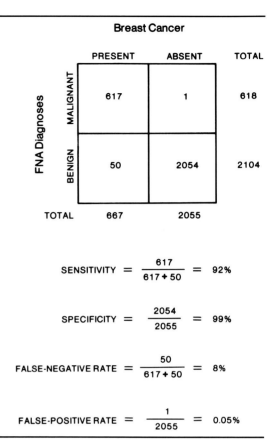

Figure 18.1.
Sensitivity and specificity of benign and malignant breast aspirates.

Based on our nine years' experience the specificity and sensitivity of the technique is shown in Figure 18.1. Please note that only diagnostic breast aspirates have been considered. Unsatisfactory and inconclusive aspirates have not been included.

INCONCLUSIVE ASPIRATES

In our cytopathology reports, under interpretation, there are four categories: (1) no evidence of cancer, (2) diagnostic of cancer, (3) unsatisfactory, and (4) other. One of these four categories has to be marked in each report. Items 1 through 3 only need a check mark. The "other" or "inconclusive" category needs a narrative description or note. Of the 247 inconclusive reports (Tables 18.3 and 18.8), 101 aspirates were diagnosed as "suspect carcinoma"; 93 aspirates were diagnosed as "atypical hyperplasia"; 48 aspirates were diagnosed as "few atypical cells, quantity not sufficient for definite diagnosis, or diagnosis deferred"; 3 aspirates were diagnosed as "suspect lymphoma"; and 2 aspirates were diagnosed as "cystosarcoma phyllodes."

Of the 101 aspirates in which we rendered a diagnosis of "suspect carcinoma," 96 cases had tissue follow-up. The histologic diagnoses were the following:

Carcinoma*	76 cases
Atypical ductal or lobular hyperplasia	8 cases
Postradiation atypia	1 case
Abscess, mastitis, or fat necrosis	3 cases
Fibrocystic disease	7 cases
Fibroadenoma	1 case

In five cases no tissue was available. Of these, one patient has been followed clinically, one patient has refused a biopsy, two patients are lost to follow-up, and one patient has died.

Of 93 aspirates diagnosed as "atypical hyperplasia," tissue follow-up was available in 68 cases. The histologic diagnoses were the following:

Carcinoma	23 cases
Lobular	6 cases
Tubular	1 case
In situ ductal	1 case
Infiltrating ductal†	15 cases
Atypical hyperplasia	8 cases
Fibroadenoma	7 cases
Fibrocystic disease	29 cases
Papilloma	1 case

No tissue was available in 25 cases. Of these, 22 patients have been followed clinically, 2 patients have been lost to follow-up, and 1 patient has died.

In those 48 aspirates in which the presence of a "few atypical cells" was reported but no definite diagnosis could be rendered, 38 patients underwent excisional biopsies. The diagnoses were:

Carcinoma	19 cases
Lobular	4 cases
Colloid	1 case
Ductal	14 cases
Atypical hyperplasia	4 cases
Fibroadenoma	3 cases
Fibrocystic disease	9 cases
Papilloma	1 case
Organizing hematoma	2 cases

*Note: Eleven patients were reaspirated by a pathologist and two by a surgeon and a definite diagnosis of carcinoma was rendered on reaspiration.

†Note: Seven of the fifteen infiltrating ductal carcinomas showed no residual tumor in the mastectomy specimen. One case was diagnosed as carcinoma on reaspiration.

No tissue was available in 10 cases. All of these patients are being followed clinically.

In the three instances in which the report indicated "suspect lymphoma," the diagnosis was confirmed histologically in two cases. The third patient expired, and we have been unable to learn the cause of death.

In two instances the cytologic diagnosis of cystosarcoma was made, but we could not establish whether it was benign or malignant in the aspirated material. Both lesions were excised. One was a malignant cystosarcoma phyllodes and the other was a cystosarcoma of "intermediate grade."

We have attempted to describe what we do and why we do it. Please remember that our success did not happen quickly. It took two years to convince the clinicians of the technique's usefulness and for us to see it begin to prosper. We constantly consider ways to improve our techniques and the quality of our diagnoses. This book describes what we are doing at present, but probably it will not be quite the same a few years from now. In addition, we wish to emphasize that what has worked for us may not work for everyone else. You will have to adapt and modify this to suit your particular circumstances. One cannot be dogmatic. If you believe that the combination of hematologic and Papanicolaou stains will help you obtain a more accurate diagnosis, then pursue that route. If you find that Millipore filter preparations are helpful and you can afford them, then use them. If you do not like to see patients but can train your surgical colleagues to provide you with good aspirates, that can be satisfactory also. It does not matter which road we travel as long as we reach our common goal of a correct diagnosis, obtained promptly and economically.

References

Abele JS, Miller TR, Goodson III WH, et al. Fine-needle aspiration of palpable breast masses. A program for staged implementation. Arch Surg 1983;118:859−863.

Agnantis NT, Rosen PP. Mammary carcinoma with osteoclast-like giant cells. A study of eight cases with follow-up data. Am J Clin Pathol 1979;72:383−389.

Azzarelli A, Guzzon A, Pilotti S, et al. Accuracy of breast cancer diagnosis by physical, radiologic and cytologic combined examinations. Tumori 1983;69:137−141.

Bell DA, Hajdu SI, Urban JA, et al. Role of aspiration cytology in the diagnosis and management of mammary lesions in office practice. Cancer 1983;51:1182−1189.

Bolmgren J, Jacobson B, Nordenström B. Stereotaxic instrument for needle biopsy of the mamma. Am J Roentgenol 1977;129:121−125.

Chu EW, Hoye RC. The clinician and the cytopathologist evaluate fine needle aspiration cytology. Acta Cytol 1973;17:413−417.

Coates MR, Pilch YH, Benfield JR. Changing concepts in establishing the diagnosis of breast masses. Am J Surg 1977;134:77−81.

Curtin CT, Pertschuk LP, Mitchell V. Histochemical determination of estrogen and progesterone binding in fine needle aspirates of breast cancer: correlation with conventional biochemical assays. Acta Cytol 1982;26:841−846.

Dixon JM, Anderson TJ, Lamb J, et al. Fine needle aspiration cytology, in relationships to clinical examination and mammography in the diagnosis of a solid breast mass. Br J Surg 1984;71:593−596.

Dupont WD, Page DL. Risk factors for breast cancer in women with proliferative breast disease. N Engl J Med 1985;312:146−151.

Elston CW, Cotton RE, Davies CJ, et al. A comparison of the use of the 'Tru-Cut' needle and fine needle aspiration cytology in the pre-operative diagnosis of carcinoma of the breast. Histopathology 1978;2:239−254.

Fahn A. Plant anatomy. New York:Pergamon Press, 1974, Second edition:108−114.

Feldman PS, Covell JL. Fine needle aspiration cytology and its clinical applications: Breast & lung. Chicago: ASCP Press, 1985.

Fisher B. Reappraisal of breast biopsy prompted by the use of lumpectomy:surgical strategy. JAMA 1985;253:3585−3588.

Foster Jr. RS. Core-cutting needle biopsy for the diagnosis of breast cancer. Am J Surg 1982;143:622−623.

Frable WJ. Thin-needle aspiration biopsy. A personal experience with 469 cases. Am J Clin Pathol 1976;65:168−182.

Frable WJ. Thin-needle aspiration biopsy. Bennington JL, series ed. Philadelphia:WB Saunders Co., 1983, Vol. 14.

Frable WJ. Needle aspiration of the breast. Cancer 1984;53:671−676.

Franzén S, Zajicek J. Aspiration biopsy in diagnosis of palpable lesions of the breast. Critical review of 3479 consecutive biopsies. Acta Radiol [Ther] (Stockholm) 1968; 7:241−262.

Fritsches HG, Muller EA. Pseudosarcomatous fasciitis of the breast. Cytologic and histologic features. Acta Cytol 1983;27:73−75.

Frost JK. The cell in health and disease. An evaluation of cellular morphologic expression of biologic behavior. Switzerland: S Karger AG, 1969:51−56.

Galblum LI, Oertel YC. Subareolar abscess of the breast: diagnosis by fine-needle aspiration. Am J Clin Pathol 1983;80:496−499.

Gallager, HS. Pathologic types of breast cancer: their prognoses. Cancer 1984;53: 623−629.

Goodwin JS, Goodwin JM. The tomato effect: rejection of highly efficacious therapies. JAMA 1984;251:2387−2390.

Gunduz N, Zheng S, Fisher B. Fluoresceinated estrone binding by cells from human breast cancers obtained by needle aspiration. Cancer 1983;52:1251−1256.

Hall FM. Screening mammography: potential problems on the horizon. N Engl J Med 1986; 314:53−55.

Homer MJ, Smith TJ, Marchant DJ. Outpatient needle localization and biopsy for nonpalpable breast lesions. JAMA 1984;252:2452−2454.

Ingram DM, Sterrett GF, Sheiner HJ, et al. Fine-needle aspiration cytology in the management of breast disease. Med J Aust 1983;2:170−173.

Jayaram G. Cytomorphology of tuberculous mastitis. A report of nine cases with fine needle aspiration cytology. Acta Cytol 1985;29:974−978.

Kehler M, Albrechtsson U. Mammographic fine needle biopsy of non-palpable breast lesions. Acta Radiol Diagnosis 1984;25:273−276.

Kern WH. The diagnosis of breast cancer by fine-needle aspiration smears. JAMA 1979;241:1125−1127.

King LS. 'Hey, you!' and other forms of address. JAMA 1985;254:266−267.

Kline TS, Joshi LP, Neal HS. Fine-needle aspiration of the breast:diagnoses and pitfalls. A review of 3545 cases. Cancer 1979;44:1458−1464.

Kline TS. Handbook of fine needle aspiration biopsy cytology. St. Louis: CV Mosby Co., 1981.

Koss LG. Thin needle aspiration biopsy. Editorial. Acta Cytol 1980;24:1−3.

Koss LG, Woyke S, Olszewski W. Aspiration biopsy. Cytologic interpretation and histologic bases. New York:Igaku−Shoin, 1984.

Lamas AM, Horwitz RI, Peck D. Usefulness of mammography in the diagnosis and management of breast disease in postmenopausal women. JAMA 1984;252:2999−3002.

Lever JV, Trott PA, Webb AJ. Fine needle aspiration cytology. J Clin Pathol 1985;38: 1−11.

Lindgren A, Sällström J, Adami H−O. Fine needle biopsy in estrogen receptor determination in breast cancer. Eur J Cancer Suppl 1980;1:67−69.

Linsk J, Kreuzer G, Zajicek J. Cytologic diagnosis of mammary tumors from aspiration biopsy smears: II. Studies on 210 fibroadenomas and 210 cases of benign dysplasia. Acta Cytol 1972;16:130−138.

Linsk JA, Franzen S. Clinical aspiration cytology. Philadephia:JB Lippincott Co., 1983.

Löwhagen T, Rubio CA. The cytology of the granular cell myoblastoma of the breast. Report of a case. Acta Cytol 1977;21:314−315.

McLean J, Sugiura K. Does aspiration biopsy of tumors cause distant metastasis? J Lab Clin Med 1937;22:1254−1257.

Magarey CJ, Watson WJ. The outpatient diagnosis of breast lumps. Aust NZ J Surg 1976;46:344−349.

Malberger E, Toledano C, Barzilai A, et al. The decisive role of fine needle aspiration cytology in the preoperative work-up of breast cancer. Isr J Med Sci 1981;17:899−904.

Marasà L, Tomasino RM. Aspiration cytology of the breast. I. Comparison of cytologic and histologic findings. Pathologica 1982;74:183−192.

Martin HE, Ellis EB. Biopsy by needle puncture and aspiration. Ann Surg 1930;92:169−181.

Martin HE, Ellis EB. Aspiration biopsy. Surg Gynecol Obstet 1934;59:578−589.

Merle S, Zajdela A, Magdelenat H. Progesterone-receptor assay in fine needle aspirates of breast tumors. Letter to the editor. Acta Cytol 1985;29:496−498.

Mühlow A. A device for precision needle biopsy of the breast at mammography. Am J Roentgenol 1974;121:843−845.

Nayar M, Saxena HMK. Tuberculosis of the breast:a cytomorphologic study of needle aspirates and nipple discharges. Acta Cytol 1984;28:325−328.

Naylor B. Pathology Department, University of Michigan Medical School. Personal Communication, Oct. 1981.

Newsome JF, McLelland R. A word of caution concerning mammography. JAMA 1986;255:528.

Nielsen M, Andersen JA, Henriksen FW, et al. Metastases to the breast from extra-mammary carcinomas. Acta Path Microbiol Scand [A] 1981;89:251−256.

Oertel YC: Fine-needle aspiration. A personal view. Lab Med 1982;13:343−347.

Oertel YC, Galblum LI. Fine needle aspiration of the breast: diagnostic criteria. Pathol Annu 1983;18:375−407.

Page DL, Dupont WD, Rogers LW, et al. Atypical hyperplastic lesions of the female breast. A long-term follow-up study. Cancer 1985;55:2698−2708.

Pettinato G, Petrella G, Manco A, et al. Carcinoma of the breast with osteoclast-like giant cells. Fine-needle aspiration cytology, histology and electron microscopy of 5 cases. Appl Pathol 1984;2:168−178.

Poulsen HS, Schultz H, Bichel P. Oestrogen-receptor determinations on fine-needle aspirations from malignant tumours of the breast. Europ J Cancer 1979;15:1431−1438.

Raff LJ. Frozen section needle biopsy of the breast: a technique of limited usefulness. Breast 1982;8:11−13.

Ragaz J, Baird R, Rebbeck P, et al. Neoadjuvant (preoperative) chemotherapy for breast cancer. Cancer 1985;56:719−724.

Rimsten A, Stenkvist B, Johanson H, et al. The diagnostic accuracy of palpation and fine-needle biopsy and an evaluation of their combined use in the diagnosis of breast lesions:report on a prospective study in 1244 women with symptoms. Ann Surg 1975;182:1−8.

Roberts JG, Preece PE, Bolton PM, et al. The 'tru-cut' biopsy in breast cancer. Clin Oncol 1975;1:297–303.

Rosen P, Hajdu SI, Robbins G, et al. Diagnosis of carcinoma of the breast by aspiration biopsy. Surg Gynecol Obstet 1972;134:837–838.

Rosen PP. Multinucleated mammary stromal giant cells:a benign lesion that simulates invasive carcinoma. Cancer 1979a;44:1305–1308.

Rosen PP. The pathological classification of human mammary carcinoma:Past, present and future. Ann Clin Lab Sci 1979b;9:144–156.

Rush MR. Fine needle aspiration biopsy:past-present-future. Lab Manage 1977;15: 33–36.

Santos GH: Should physicians be paid for their technical failures? Letter to the editor. N Engl J Med 1983;308:289.

Sattin RW, Rubin GL, Webster LA, et al. Family history and the risk of breast cancer JAMA 1985;253:1908–1913.

Schnitt SJ, Connolly JL, Harris JR, et al. Radiation-induced changes in the breast. Hum Pathol 1984;15:545–550.

Schöndorf H. Aspiration cytology of the breast. Schneider V, trans. Philadelphia:WB Saunders Co., 1978.

Shabot MM, Goldberg IM, Schick P, et al. Aspiration cytology is superior to Tru-Cut® needle biopsy in establishing the diagnosis of clinically suspicious breast masses. Ann Surg 1982;196:122–126.

Sickles EA, Klein DL, Goodson WH, et al. Mammography after needle aspiration of palpable breast masses. Am J Surg 1983;145:395–397.

Snyder RE, Rosen P. Radiography of breast specimens. Cancer 1971;28:1608–1611.

Söderström N. Fine-needle aspiration biopsy. Used as a direct adjunct in clinical diagnostic work. New York: Grune & Stratton, 1966.

Stewart FW. The diagnosis of tumors by aspiration. Am J Pathol 1933;9:801–812.

Strawbridge HTG, Bassett AA, Foldes I. Role of cytology in management of lesions of the breast. Surg Gynecol Obstet 1981;152:1–7.

Sullivan Jr. WA. Early detection of breast cancer. Letter to the editor. JAMA 1985; 253:2195.

Svane G. Stereotaxic needle biopsy of non-palpable breast lesions:a clinical and radiologic follow-up. Acta Radiol Diagnosis 1983;24:385–390.

Svane G, Silfverswärd C. Stereotaxic needle biopsy of non-palpable breast lesions: cytologic and histopathologic findings. Acta Radiol Diagnosis 1983;24:283–288.

Thomas JM, Fitzharris BM, Redding WH, et al. Clinical examination, xeromammography, and fine-needle aspiration cytology in diagnosis of breast tumours. Br Med J 1978;2:1139–1141.

Vassilakos P. Tuberculosis of the breast:cytologic findings with fine-needle aspiration. A case clinically and radiologically mimicking carcinoma. Acta Cytol 1973;17:160–165.

Vickery EL. Our art, our heritage. JAMA 1983;250:913–915.

Webb AJ. Through a glass darkly (the development of needle aspiration biopsy). Bristol Med Chir J 1974;89:59–68.

Wilson SL, Ehrmann RL. The cytologic diagnosis of breast aspirations. Acta Cytol 1978;22:470–475.

Zajdela A, Ghossein NA, Pilleron JP, et al. The value of aspiration cytology in the diagnosis of breast cancer: experience at the Fondation Curie. Cancer 1975;35:499–506.

Zajicek J. Aspiration biopsy cytology, Part 1, Cytology of supradiaphragmatic organs. Wied GL, ed. Switzerland: S Karger AG, 1974, Vol. 4.

Index

Abscess, 71, 171, 185. *See also* Mastitis
Accessory mammary tissue, 89
Adenocarcinoma, 112–149. *See also* Ductal adenocarcinoma; Lobular carcinoma; *specific types*
Adenoid cystic carcinoma, 127–130
Adequate samples, 30
Adipose tissue, 34–36
Age
  and atypical ductal hyperplasia, 101, 102
  and fibroadenoma, 176
Air-drying artifacts, 8–9
Albuminized slides, 18
Anesthesia, 19
Apocrine carcinoma, 124–126
Apocrine metaplastic cells, 38–41
Artifacts, 49–55
Aspirates
  adequate, 30
  inconclusive, 194–196
  occasional contents of, 45–55
  unsatisfactory, 31–32, 187
  usual contents of, 34–44
Aspiration
  advantages and disadvantages of, 4–6
  vs. biopsy, 1, 7
  complications of, 7
  consistency of lesion on, 184
  equipment for, 16–19
  guidelines for, 185
  history of, 3
  of nonpalpable lesions, 3, 182–183
  number performed per year, 2
  pain with, 91
  pitfalls of, 167–181

statistical summary of, 187–196
  success at, 29–33, 186
  technique for, 19–22
  training for, 28
Aspiration room, 13–14
Aspiration team, 12–13
Aspir Gun, 17
Atypia, radiation-induced, 179–180
Atypical ductal hyperplasia, 94–103
Atypical fibroadenoma, 176–178
Axillary mammary tissue, 89, 166
Axillary masses, 33, 89, 164, 166
Axillary metastases, 30, 161–162

Bacterial diseases, 71–76
Benign neoplasms, 78–89
  calcifications in, 49
  fibroadenoma, 30, 38, 78–83
  granular cell myoblastoma, 84–88, 168
  lipoma, 83
  neurilemoma, 165–166
  nodular fasciitis, 88–89
  papilloma, 83–86
  schwannoma, 165–166
Benign non-neoplasias, 56–78
  abscess, 71
  comedomastitis, 57, 64–66
  cysts, 32, 56
  ductal ectasia, 57, 62, 63, 168–169
  ductal hyperplasia, 57–59, 94–103
  fat necrosis, 68, 69, 162, 170–171
  fatty replacement, 64, 83
  fibrocystic disease, 56

fibrous mastopathy, 30, 64
gynecomastia, 91–93
hematoma, 68–70, 167–168
herpesvirus, 74, 76–78
lactation, 68–71
lymph node, intramammary, 89–91
mastitis, acute, 71–72
mastitis granulomatous, 74–76
sclerosing adenosis, 57
squamous metaplasia, 57, 59–62
subareolar abscess, 71, 73
Biopsy. *See* Needle biopsy
Bipolar nuclei, 38, 82
Blood vessels, in malignancy, 111
  in colloid carcinoma, 118–119
Blunt branching, 78, 81
Breast lobules, 44

Calcifications, 49
  apocrine carcinoma, 125
  carcinoma with giant cells, 137, 140
Cameco Syringe Pistol, 17
Carcinoma
  adenoid cystic, 127–130, 184, 185
  apocrine, 124–126
  with carcinoid features, 129, 135–136
  colloid, 115–121
  comedo, 113–115
  consistency of, 184
  diagnostic criteria for, 104–111
  ductal, 103, 112–145
  in fibroadenoma, 82
  infiltrating, 112–113
  inflammatory, 128–129, 133–134

201

lobular, 145–149, 161
male, 149
medullary, 121–124
with multinucleated giant cells, 137–140
with necrosis, 113–115
Paget's disease, 143–145
papillary, 115–117
with pregnancy, 149
recurrent, 161–163, 179
renal cell, 158–160
squamous cell, 140–142
tubular, 127–128, 130–132
unsuspected, 5
Cardiopulmonary resuscitation, 13
Cells
apocrine metaplastic, 38
bipolar nuclei, 38
ductal, 34, 37–39
histiocytic, 39, 42
myoepithelial, 37–38, 92
squamous metaplastic, 57, 59–62
Cellular fragility in
carcinoid-like carcinoma, 129
granular cell tumor, 84, 168
lymphoma, 150
Cellulose fibers, 51, 53, 54
Cholesterol crystals, 69, 70, 143
Colloid carcinoma, 115–121, 184, 185
Comedocarcinoma, 64, 113–115, 185
Comedomastitis, 57, 64–66, 171, 185
Costs, 4, 6
Cover glass, 18–19
Crystals
cholesterol, 69, 70, 143
fernlike, 51
oleic acid, 42, 44
Cystosarcoma phyllodes, 154–155, 175
Cysts, 32, 56
Cytotechnologist, 12

Diagnostic criteria for carcinoma, 104–111
Diff-Quik
advantages and disadvantages, 9, 10
and nuclear changes, 108
vs. Papanicolaou's stain, 8–10, 25
Ductal adenocarcinoma, 103, 112–145, 185

vs. atypical ductal hyperplasia, 103
consistency of, 184
diagnostic criteria for, 9, 104–111
vs. fibroadenoma, 174
infiltrating, 112–113
male, 149
with pregnancy, 149
Ductal cells, 34, 37–39
Ductal ectasia, 57, 62, 63, 168–169
Ductal hyperplasia, 57–59, 94–103

Ectasia, ductal, 57, 62, 63, 168–169
Equipment, 16–18
Estrogen receptors, 6
Excisional biopsy
for atypical hyperplasia, 101–103
granulomata following, 74

False negative results, 6, 186, 190–194
False positive results, 6, 78, 167–168, 190–194
Fat necrosis, 68, 69, 162, 170–171, 185
Fatty replacement, 64, 83, 184
Fernlike crystals, 51
Fibroadenoma, 30, 38, 78–83, 174–178, 185
vs. adenocarcinoma, 174
atypical, 176–178
consistency of, 184
vs. cystosarcoma, 175
in elderly women, 176
vs. fibrocystic disease, 82–83
intranuclear inclusions in, 82
in pregnancy, 175–176
Fibroadipose tissue, 36
Fibrocystic disease, 56, 64, 185
vs. apocrine carcinoma, 124
vs. fibroadenoma, 82–83
vacuoles in, 108
Fibrous mastopathy, 30, 64, 67, 184
Fine needle aspiration. See Aspiration

Giant cells, multinucleated. See Multinucleated giant cells
Glass slides, 18–19
Granular cell tumor, 84–88, 168
Granulomatous mastitis, 74–76
Gynecomastia, 91–93

Hemacytometer, 18–19
Hematologic stains, 8–10
Hematoma, 68–70, 167–168, 185
Herpesvirus infection, 74, 76–78, 162, 167
Histiocytes, 39, 42
Hormonal changes, 68–71
Hospitals, 6
Hyperplasia, ductal, 57–59, 94–103

Inconclusive aspirates, 194–196
Infiltrating carcinoma, 108, 112–113
Inflammatory carcinoma, 128–129, 133–134
Informed consent, 11
Intranuclear inclusions, 82, 108, 156

Lactation, 68, 70, 71
Lesion, consistency, 184
Leukemia, 150–152, 185
Lipoma, 30, 83, 184
Lobular carcinoma, 145–149, 161, 184, 185
Lumina, 109
Lymph nodes
intramammary, 89–91
metastases to, 161–164
Lymphoma, 150–151

Malignant neoplasms
and age, 30
calcifications in, 49, 125, 137, 140
diagnostic criteria for, 104–111
ductal carcinoma, 104–111, 112–115
metastatic to axilla, 161–162
metastatic to breast, 156–160
nonepithelial, 150–155
nonpalpable, 182–183
seeding of, 181
Mammogram, 33, 101, 103, 183
after aspiration, 20
Mastectomy, 103, 161, 186
without frozen section, 193
Mastitis, 7, 71, 74, 171, 185
acute, 71, 72, 171–173
granulomatous, 74–76
May-Grünwald Giemsa stain, 8
Medullary carcinoma, 121–124, 184
Melanoma, 108, 111, 156–158, 185

Menses, 89, 101
Metastases
  axillary, 89, 161–162
  chest wall, 161–163
Metastatic tumors
  in breast, 156–160
  melanoma, 108, 111, 156–158, 185
  renal cell, 158–160, 185
Microcalcifications, 49, 125, 137, 140
Mitoses, 111
Multinucleated giant cells in
  carcinoma, 137–140
  ductal ectasia, 57, 63, 168
  fibroadenoma, 177–178
  granulomata, 74–75
  hematoma, 68
  herpesvirus, 77–78
Mycosis fungoides, 150–153
Myoepithelial cells, 37–38, 92

Necrosis, 113–115
Needle biopsy
  advantages and disadvantages, 7
  vs. aspiration, 1, 7
Needles, 1, 2, 18, 19
Neoplasms
  of nervous tissue, 165–166
  See also Benign neoplasms;
    Malignant neoplasms
Nervous tissue, neoplasms of, 165–166
Neurilemoma, 33, 165–166
Nodular fasciitis, 88–89
Nonpalpable lesions, 182–183
Nuclei
  bipolar, 38, 82
  in carcinoma, 104, 108
  pleomorphic, 104, 114
  staining of, 108
  stripped, 38, 82
Nucleoli in, 108
  apocrine cells, 39
  granular cell tumor, 84
  lactation, 68
  medullary carcinoma, 123
  metastatic melanoma, 156

Oleic acid crystals, 42, 44

Osmotic effect, 51

Paget's disease, 143–145
Pain, 91
Palpable masses, management of, 14
Palpatory ability, 13
Papanicolaou's stain, 8–10, 25
  advantages and disadvantages
    of, 9, 10
  and nuclear changes, 108
Papillary carcinoma, 115–117, 185
Papilloma, 83–86
Papillomatosis, 57, 94–103
Pathologist, 6, 13, 29
Patient
  advantages of aspiration to, 4–5
  consent of, 11
  positioning of, 186
Pitfalls, 167–181
Platelets, 45, 48
Pneumothorax, 7
Positioning the patient, 186
Postradiation atypia, 179–180
Pregnancy
  and aspiration, 5
  and axillary mass changes, 89
  and ductal carcinoma, 149
  and fibroadenoma, 175–176
Progesterone receptors, 6

Radiation-induced atypia, 179–180
Recurrent carcinoma, 161–163, 179
Renal cell carcinoma, 158–160, 185
Reusable Syringe Holder, 17

Samples, 30, 185–186
Schwannoma, 33, 165–166
Sclereids, 52–55
Sclerosing adenosis, 57
Secretary, 12
Seeding of tumor, 181
Self-examination, 29
Skeletal muscle, 45–47
Skin, 45, 47
Slides, 18–19

Smears
  appearance of, 185
  guidelines for exam, 185
  preparation of, 22–27
  staining of, 8–10, 25–28
Specimens
  satisfactory, 30
  unsatisfactory, 31–32, 187
Squamous cell carcinoma, 140–142
Squamous metaplasia, 57, 59–62
Staining
  and nuclear changes, 108
  precipitate, 49
  smears, 8–10, 25–28
Stains
  Diff-Quik, 8–10
  hematologic, 8–10
  May-Grünwald Giemsa, 8
  Papanicolaou, 8–10
  precipitates of, 49, 50
Starch granules, 52, 54, 55
Stone cells, 52–55
Stripped nuclei, 38, 82
Subareolar abscess, 71, 73, 185
Surgeon, 5
Syringe holder, 16–17
Syringes, 18

Technique, 16–28
Thoracic wall recurrence, 161–166
Thyroid aspirates, 31
Thyroid carcinoma, 108
Training, 28
Trauma, 68
True cut biopsy. See Needle
  biopsy
Tuberculosis, 74–76
Tubular carcinoma, 127–128, 130–132
Tumors
  granular cell, 84–88, 168
  See also Benign neoplasms;
    Malignant neoplasms; Meta-
    static tumors
Tumor cellularity, 104

Vacuoles, 108, 148
Viral diseases, 74–78